Swiss Ball

For Total Fitness

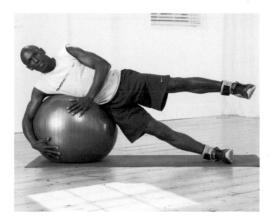

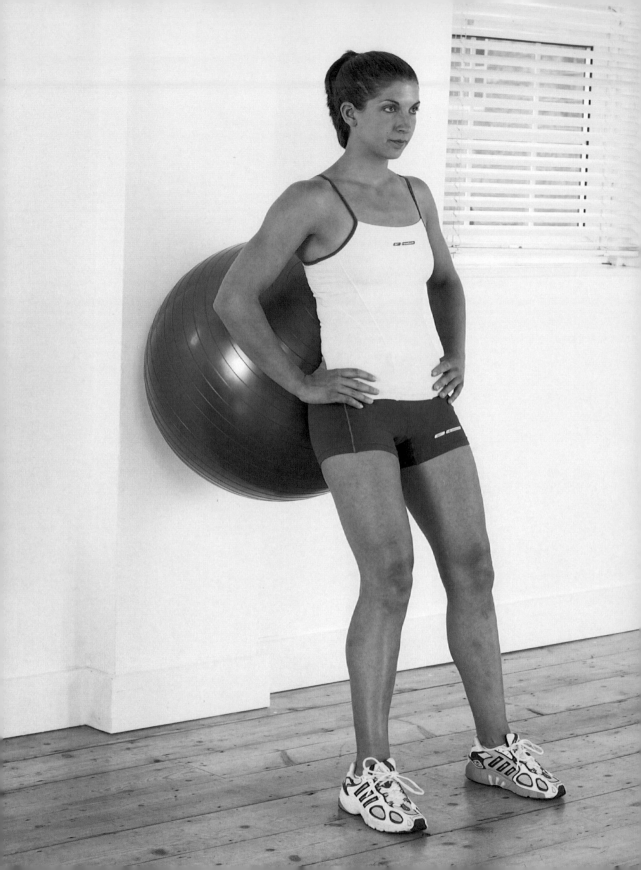

Swiss Ball
For Total Fitness

A STEP-BY-STEP GUIDE

IMPROVE STRENGTH & STABILITY

20-MINUTE WORKOUTS

James Milligan

Main Street
A division of Sterling Publishing Co., Inc.
New York

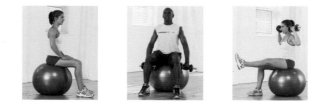

Library of Congress Cataloging-in-Publication Data Available

10 9 8 7 6 5 4 3 2

Published by Main Street a division of Sterling Publishing Co., Inc.
387 Park Avenue South, New York, NY 10016
© 2004 by PRC Publishing
An imprint of **Chrysalis** Books Group plc

Distributed in Canada by Sterling Publishing
c/o Canadian Manda Group, 165 Dufferin Street
Toronto, Ontario, Canada M6K 3H6

1 4027 1965 5

For information about custom editions, special sales, premium and
corporate purchases, please contact Sterling Special Sales
Department at 800-805-5489 or specialsales@sterlingpub.com

Contents

Introduction

The term "Swiss Ball" was given to this fantastically versatile piece of equipment by physiotherapists in the United States during the late 1980s when it began to be used for physical therapy and rehabilitation from injury. It was named the "Swiss Ball" as it was first used in Switzerland, though the ball was actually manufactured by an Italian plastics company in 1963. The Swiss Ball is now widely used around the world, in everything from light aerobics classes to professional athletic training institutions, as more and more people learn the benefits of using this simple yet highly effective training aid.

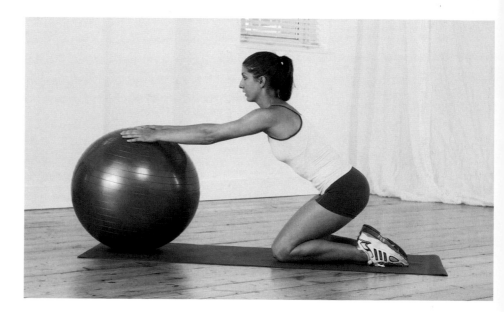

What makes Swiss Balls so good?

We all need to be balanced and stable. Even when sat at a desk all day, stability is required to hold a correct posture. A lack of balance and stability around your joints can lead to injury and referred complaints such as back and neck pain. Effective muscle proprioception (communication with the brain resulting in muscle action) is vital in maintaining balance and stability, especially in sport. The nature and instability of a ball when a body rests against it, makes it the perfect training tool. It helps to improve your center of balance and at the same time strengthen your "core."

All muscles work together in a synergistic chain; by following the exercises and progressions in this book you will learn to create improved balance, stability, and even strength and muscle tone, maximizing the efficiency of this chain. Your muscle control and coordination will be greatly improved, as the instability of the ball requires you to concentrate on your balance as well as the movement that you are performing. Even more important, a Swiss Ball will add fun and variety to your fitness training routine.

Additional benefits of using a Swiss Ball

Low cost

Swiss Balls provide training without the use of expensive equipment, or the need to join a gym. For the price of less than a month's gym membership, you can set yourself up with all that you need for a complete Swiss Ball workout.

Light weight

Unlike other training equipment that would be required to complete some of the exercises shown in this book, the Swiss Ball is light in weight, making it easier and safer to move around.

Storage and portability

Because the Swiss Ball is lightweight and compact when deflated, it does not require much storage space, unlike bulky frames and benches. This also means that you can take it with you anywhere you go, which is especially beneficial for those who travel regularly, as it enables you to maintain the consistency of your exercise program.

Time efficiency

You can plan your time more efficiently by using a Swiss Ball, as you won't need to work around gym schedules or allow for additional traveling time. You can pick it up whenever you want and wherever you are.

What results can you expect from using a Swiss Ball?

- Enhanced balance, stability, and control of deep muscle tissues
- Improved posture and support around joints
- Greater muscle strength, power, and endurance
- Greater flexibility and range of movement in joints
- Improved metabolism, body weight control, and energy
- Greater enjoyment of everyday activities and sports
- Prevention of muscle and joint atrophy (loss of muscle mass) caused by aging
- Reduced risk of injury

The terminology of the anatomy and muscle groups being worked in each section has been kept to a level where it is easily understandable for a beginner, yet is still informative to those who have good basic knowledge of other training methods. It is outside the remit of this book to go into great anatomical detail, but the guide to muscle areas on pages 10 and 11 is an excellent start to understanding the muscle areas you will be working on.

Safety Precautions

Before commencing any exercise with a Swiss Ball, please ensure you have checked the following:

1. Condition of ball

Examine the Swiss Ball before each use, checking for stress marks and punctures. Purchase an anti-burst ball, designed to take up to 300kg in weight. Always take note of the manufacturers' recommendations with regard to its resistance to weight.

2. Ball size and inflation

To check that you have the right size ball for your body size and that it is inflated correctly, sit on top and in the center of the Swiss Ball. Your hips should be level or slightly higher than your knees, with them ideally flexed to a 90-degree angle, and your feet flat on the floor. Follow the manufacturers' instructions for optimal inflation.

3. Ball storage

Swiss Balls should be stored at room temperature. Do not store the ball in cold temperatures as this can have a negative effect on its expansion properties.

4. Exercise area suitability

Give yourself plenty of free space to perform the exercises. Choose an area of flooring that is non-slip with nothing in close proximity that you could fall onto.

Correct and safe usage

- Make sure that you understand how to do each exercise properly by carefully reading through and following the full instructions before starting your workout. Improper use can cause serious injury.
- Wear appropriate clothing, ensuring that it is not too baggy or slippery. Use footwear that has a sole with good grip.
- When using weights, be cautious. Remember that the ball will be unstable, making the weights harder to manage.
- Allow sufficient rest periods (48 hours) between workouts for recovery and to prevent over training.
- If you are new to Swiss Ball training it is advisable to build up the exercise intensity and frequency gradually. The 20-minute routines will take you through the progressions of using a Swiss Ball, however, it is not advisable to start with one of the advanced routines until you have built up a good foundation with the beginner routines.
- It is advisable to have someone with you to assist your balance at first when progressing to the more advanced stability exercises.

Health

- If you are not used to exercise or have a medical condition, please check with your physician/ doctor before commencing any form of exercise.

Equipment

For the exercises in this book you will require the following equipment:

1. Swiss Ball
There are many types and sizes of Swiss Ball available. Follow the individual manufacturer's guidelines to choose the correct size for you. Also ensure that you purchase a hand pump. Do not use an electrically operated pump.

2. Free weights
Dumbbells are available in various guises. Some are fixed weight and others are adjustable. Choose a variety from a few kilos upward.

3. Ankle weights
Ankle weights are an ideal way to add resistance against the movement of a limb, and come in a variety of weights. Choose a medium weight for the exercises in this book.

4. Medicine ball
Medicine balls are easy and comfortable to hold, and are available in various resistance levels.

5. Exercise mat
If you are exercising on a shiny surface or a hard wood floor, it would be advisable to use a mat for grip and comfort.

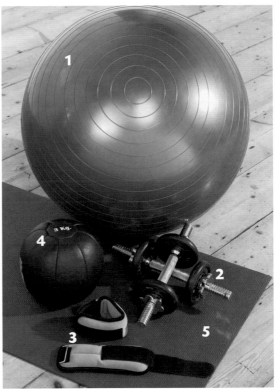

How to choose the correct size of Swiss Ball

The following sizes should be used as a general guide:

HEIGHT	BALL SIZE REQUIRED
Up to 5' 6"	55 cm (22 in.)
5' 7" – 6' 0"	65 cm (26 in.)
6' 1" – 6' 9"	75 cm (30 in.)

Please note that each manufacturer will provide their own size guidelines; so be sure to follow their individual recommendations.

Muscle Areas

To provide you with a better understanding of the location of areas that are being worked please refer to the following diagrams. Main muscle group names are listed for each exercise.

Major anterior muscle groups

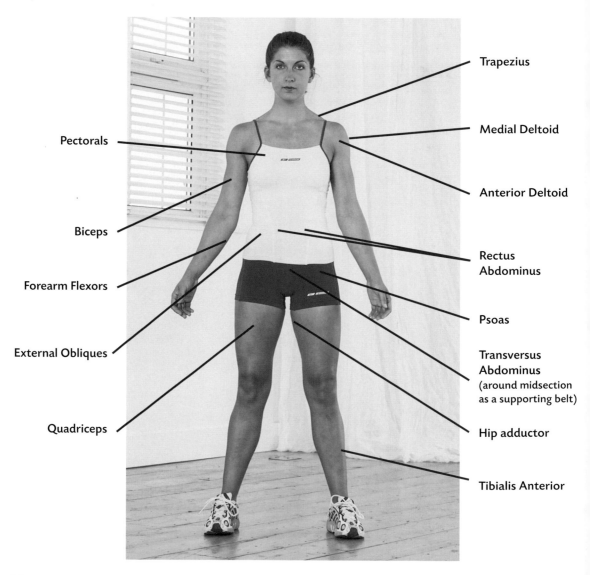

Trapezius

Medial Deltoid

Anterior Deltoid

Pectorals

Rectus
Abdominus

Biceps

Forearm Flexors

Psoas

External Obliques

Transversus
Abdominus
(around midsection
as a supporting belt)

Quadriceps

Hip adductor

Tibialis Anterior

Major posterior muscle groups

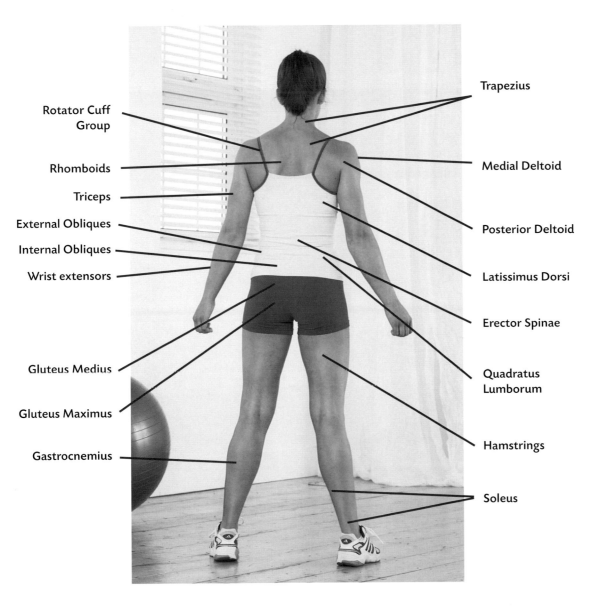

Rotator Cuff Group

Rhomboids

Triceps

External Obliques

Internal Obliques

Wrist extensors

Gluteus Medius

Gluteus Maximus

Gastrocnemius

Trapezius

Medial Deltoid

Posterior Deltoid

Latissimus Dorsi

Erector Spinae

Quadratus Lumborum

Hamstrings

Soleus

Activating and Holding the Correct Posture

To perform the exercises within this book correctly and safely, it is important that you learn how to position your body in neutral alignment. Finding this alignment will increase the effectiveness of the exercise by activating the abdominal and pelvic stabilizing muscles used to form a supportive girdle around the lower back.

Neutral alignment is when all major joints (or selected joints, depending on the exercise) are in line with one another. For example, your body and legs would be neutrally aligned when you can draw a straight line from your shoulder to your ankles passing through your hips and knees.

To help you hold a neutral position and compensate for the instability of the ball, you require support from the core muscle groups. You will see references to the "core" throughout this book. The core muscles are stabilizers that have very deep attachments to their access of movement. For example, the Transversus Abdominus has a stabilizing role in preventing your pelvis from tilting while in a bridge position with legs straight. The main aim of activating your core when doing exercises using the Swiss Ball is to effectively recruit the midsection musculature, learning to control the position of the lower back during the various dynamic movements used in this book.

Your stabilizing muscles will be stressed to a variety of intensities with each exercise. You can control the instability to a degree by altering the inflation of the ball. If the ball is fully inflated and more solid it will require greater stability than if it was softer, forming a wider contact area with the floor.

Here are some examples of the neutral alignment and correct postures that you will need to master:

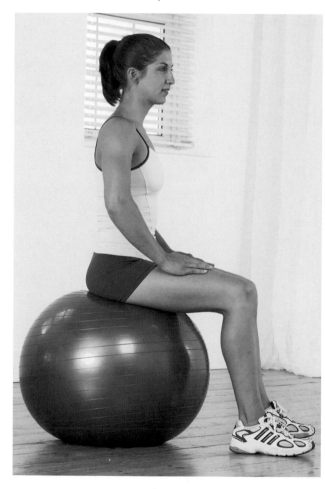

seated on the ball

1 Place yourself directly in the center of the Swiss Ball.
2 Sit on the ball with your feet flat on the floor.
3 Knees should be bent to 90 degrees.
4 Activate and tighten your abdominal muscles to support and straighten your midsection.
5 Keep your eyes fixed straight ahead so that your neck is straight.
6 Hold your torso vertical and neutrally aligned from shoulders to hips.

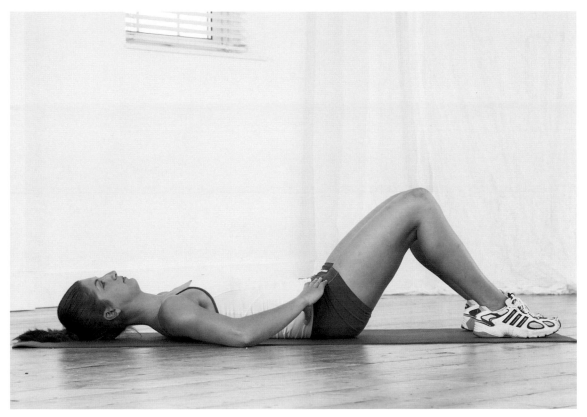

lying on the floor

1 Lie on your back on the floor with your knees bent and feet flat on the floor.
2 Pull your navel in, imagining that you are trying to get it to the floor as you tighten your lower abdominal muscles.
3 Place your finger tips either side of your lower abdominals so that you can feel them flatten and tighten as you pull your abdominals in.
4 Keep your back flat on the floor from your shoulders to your pelvis, making sure that there is no arch in the small of your back.
5 Continue to breathe normally as you hold your abdominal muscles tight.

reverse bridge position

1 Lie on your back on top of the ball with your knees bent at 90 degrees.
2 The ball should be positioned so that it sits directly between your shoulder blades.
3 Place your feet shoulder width apart.
4 Activate and tighten your abdominal muscles to maintain a neutral alignment, forming a straight line from your shoulders to your knees.
5 Do not to let your pelvis drop and move out of alignment.
6 Place your hands on your hips and fingers on the lower abdominals to feel that they are engaged and to maintain symmetry and balance in your upper body.

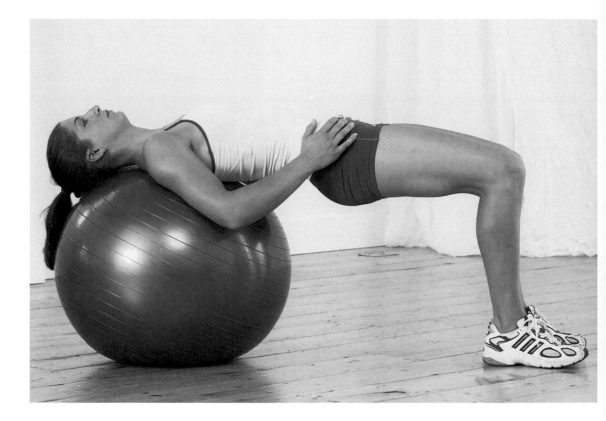

grip positions

Throughout the exercise descriptions in this book, references will be made to the different grip positions required when using weights. They are as follows:

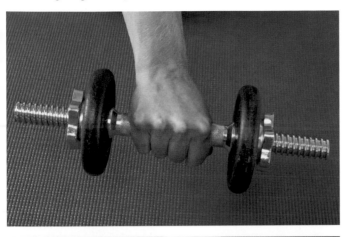

Over hand grip

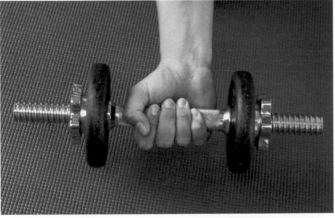

Under hand grip

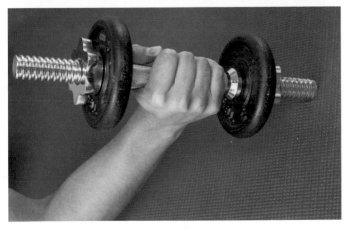

Palm inward grip

Gaining Balance and Familiarity

Beginner

lying on the ball

The first stage in familiarizing yourself with the Swiss Ball is to practice lying on it.

1 Start by lying on top of the ball with fingers and toes touching the floor for stability.

2 Shift your body weight from your toes to your fingers, rolling the ball back and forth.

3 Now try shifting your weight from side to side, touching your toes and fingers on one side, then rolling over to toes and fingers on the other side.

4 Finally, try finding your center of balance on the ball by lifting fingers and toes off the floor.

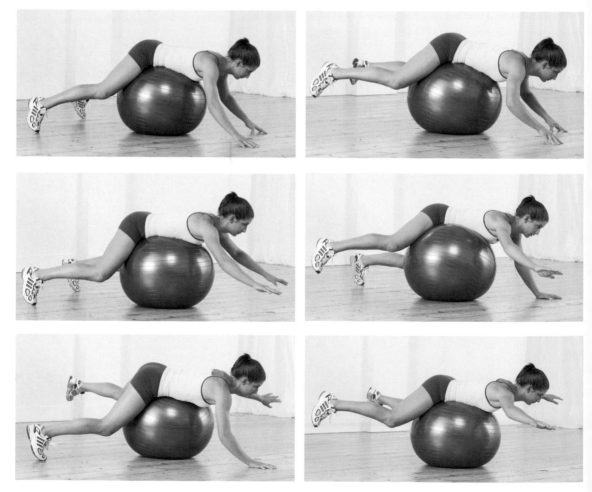

Intermediate

sitting on the ball

The second stage in finding your center of balance is to practice sitting on the Swiss Ball.

1 Sit on the center of the ball.

2 Lift your feet off the floor, and raise your arms out in front of you. Start with one leg at a time and progress to both legs. You'll be amazed how quickly you are able to tune your balance and become stable on the ball.

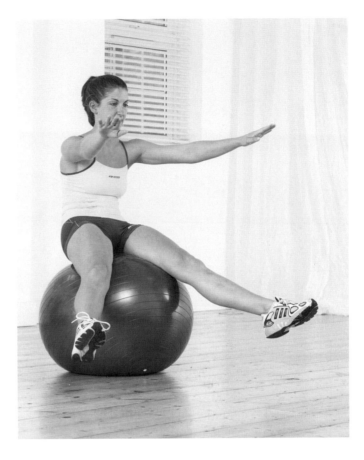

Advanced

kneeling on the ball

The third stage of learning the feel of the Swiss Ball is to practice kneeling on it. This stage requires all of your concentration to master the balance. Place a chair next to you so that you can use it to aid your balance initially.

1 Start by placing your hands on the ball, and then rest your left knee on top of the ball.

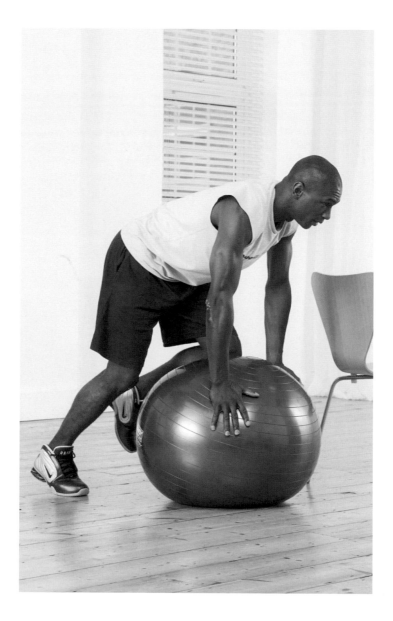

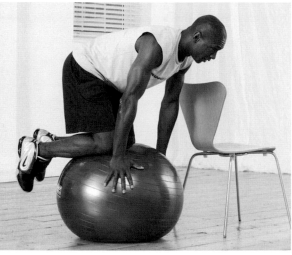

2 Lift your right leg and place your knee on top of the ball in line with your left knee. Spend some time in this position to learn the balance

3 Once you have found your balance with both hands and knees on the ball, slowly lift your hands away, and shoulders up until your torso is vertical. Use the chair next to you to hold onto initially as you develop perfect balance. Activate and tighten your abdominal muscles to hold a neutral and stable position.

Warm Up/Cool Down

Performing a warm up prior to strenuous exercise of any kind is crucial. A warm up with light aerobic and flexibility exercises is important because it:

• Prepares the muscles and joints for the activity ahead by increasing blood flow and muscle temperature.

• Reduces the risk of injury to muscles, tendons, and ligaments by making them more pliable, allowing you to move through a full range of motion more safely and effectively.

• Encourages circulation to the muscles, heart, and lungs by raising the flow of blood. This increased blood volume helps supply muscles with additional oxygen and nutrients required for exercise.

• Allows you to get into the right frame of mind through increased central nervous system function, helping you enhance factors such as muscle control and coordination, which are essential when using a Swiss Ball.

An exercise warm up should last at least 15 minutes and should focus on all areas of the body. This should start with light but brisk aerobic style movements that work large muscle group areas together. Once this has been achieved your muscles will be more pliable and ready for the flexibility exercise phase of your warm up.

These exercises can also be used at the end of your workout as a cool down phase. When performing any strenuous exercise your muscles tend to shorten with some of the fibres staying more contracted than normal. Performing flexibility exercises after your workout will help to correct and further improve muscle length, which will also aid recovery.

jogging on the spot

Areas Worked: A great warm up starting point using the large muscle groups in your legs.

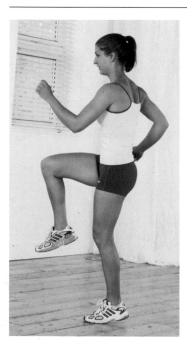

1 Lift alternate legs, pushing off your toes and flexing your knees.

2 Swing your arms back and forth in an opposite order to your legs.

Technique

• Bend your elbows to 90 degrees and lift your hands high as you swing your arms.

• Keep your eyes fixed straight ahead so that your neck is in a neutral position.

• Activate and tighten your abdominal muscles to help maintain a neutral alignment.

Hints & Tips

• Progressively increase the speed of your steps and the height of your knees.

• Control your breathing with your steps. For example, breathe in for 5 steps and out for 5 steps.

seated bounce on ball

Areas Worked: All the main muscle groups in your legs and core.

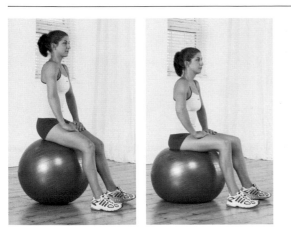

1 Sit on the ball with your feet flat on the floor. Push through your heels and extend your hips and knees slightly as if you are about to stand up.

2 Relax your legs before you lose contact with the Swiss Ball, sinking back into it. Repeat this movement for 2 to 3 minutes, or as long as desired.

Technique

- Place yourself directly in the centre of the Swiss Ball.
- Start with your knees bent to 90 degrees.
- Sit straight with your abdominal muscles activated and tightened.
- Keep your eyes fixed straight ahead so that your neck and back are neutrally aligned.
- Relax your arms and rest your hands on your thighs. Avoid using them to assist the lift.

Hints & Tips

- Progressively increase the speed and height of the bounce to enhance the warm up intensity.

seated leg rotations

Areas Worked: Warm up and mobility for the muscles in front of, and surrounding, the hip.

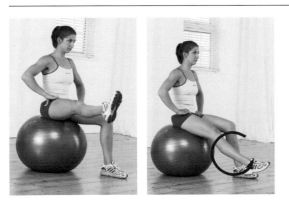

1 Sit on the ball with your feet flat on the floor. Extend one leg at the hip and knee so that it is straight.

2 Rotate your extended leg at the hip moving it in so that your foot passes the central line of your body, moves down towards the floor, and then up and out to the side. Repeat this movement for 8 to 10 repetitions.

Technique

- Place yourself directly in the centre of the Swiss Ball.
- The leg on the side that you are not working should be bent to 90 degrees at the knee, and your foot flat on the floor.
- Your extended leg should stay straight for the whole movement.
- Keep your eyes fixed straight ahead and avoid leaning your shoulders forwards when lifting the leg.
- Relax your arms and rest your hands on your hips.

Hints & Tips

- Sit straight with abdominal muscles activated and tightened.
- Progressively increase the size of the circles.

shadow boxing strides

Areas Worked: Total body warm up for all major upper and lower body muscle groups, and to switch on your coordination.

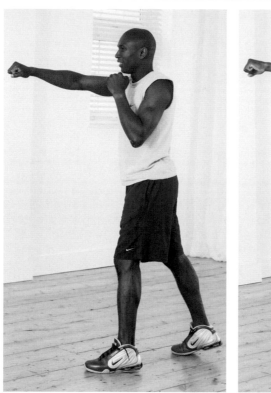 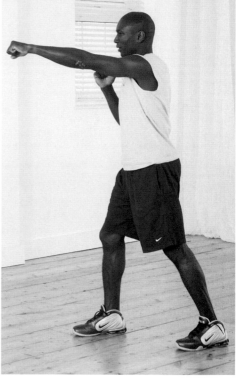

1 Stand on the spot with your left leg forward, right leg back, right arm forward, and left arm back.

2 Push off your toes and swap over the position of your feet striding the right leg forward, at the same time swap arms punching your left arm forward. Continue the alternate action for 2–3 minutes or as long as desired.

Technique

- Move your arms purposefully when punching, keeping your hands at shoulder height.
- Keep your chin up and your eyes fixed straight ahead.
- Tighten your abdominal muscles to help maintain control of your midsection.

Hints & Tips

- Keeping your weight light on your toes will enable you to use a more brisk and flowing movement.
- Gradually increase the speed of your strides and punches.
- Control your breathing with your strides. For example, breathe in for 4 strides and out for 4 strides.

ball and raise reach

Areas Worked: A good final warm up exercise that includes a full body stretch.

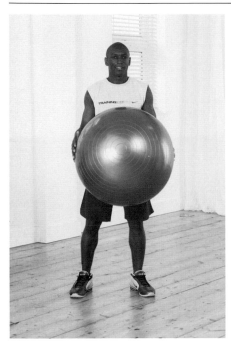

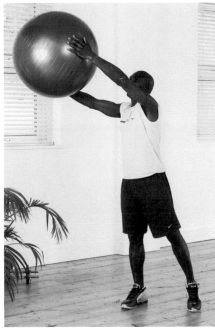

1 Stand holding the Swiss Ball in front of you.

2 Swing the ball out to the right and up, placing your weight on your right foot. Lower the ball back to the centre with your weight on both feet.

3 Swing the ball out to the left and up, now placing your weight on your left foot. Continue to swing to each side for 10–15 repetitions.

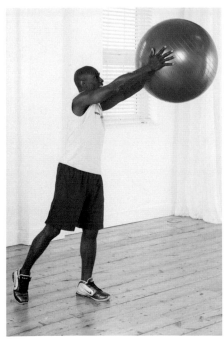

Technique

- Fully extend your arm and reach as far as possible to achieve a full stretch.
- Your legs should be straight with each reach.
- Keep your eyes fixed on the ball throughout the movement.

Hints & Tips

- Manage your breathing so that you breathe out each time you stretch out and up, and breathe in when the ball returns to the centre.

Midsection Stretches

spinal flexion and extension

Areas Worked: The length of your vertebrae, from neck to pelvis
Name of Main Muscle Group: Erector Spinae

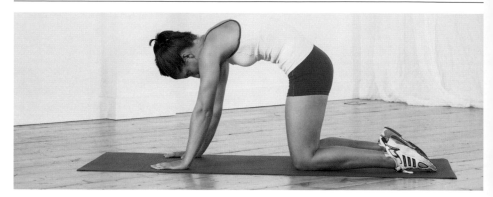

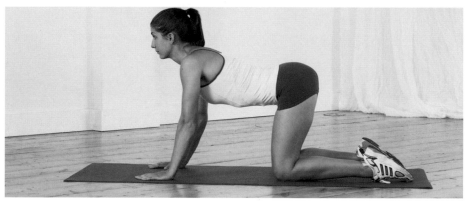

1 Position yourself on your hands and knees so that your arms and thighs are vertical. Tuck your chin in and tilt your pelvis back so that you are flexing your back and creating an arc.

2 Lift your head and tilt your pelvis forward so that you are extending your back and creating a dip. Hold the top of each movement for 3 seconds then repeat for 6 repetitions.

Technique

- Keep your hands and knees fixed in position.
- Lift the centre of your back as high as possible when flexing as if it is being lifted by a crane.
- When extending your back do so through as large a range as possible but ensuring that it is pain free.

Hints & Tips

- Relax your abdominal muscles when extending your back.
- Focus on your breathing. Breathe out when flexing and breathe in when extending.

ball reach and back flex

Areas Worked: The length of your vertebrae, from neck to pelvis and between shoulder blades
Name of Main Muscle Groups: Erector Spinae and Rhomboids

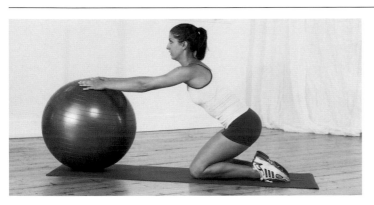

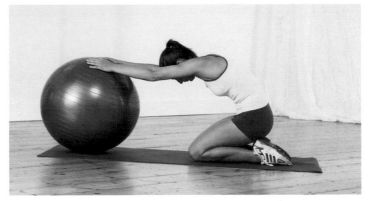

1 Kneel down with the Swiss Ball at arms length in front of you. Extend your arms out and place your hands on the top of the ball.

2 Drop your head between your shoulders and slowly sit back onto your heels. Flex your back, arching it outward as much as possible so that you feel a stretch along the length of your back. Hold this position for 15–20 seconds, and then relax.

Technique

- Keep your arms stretched out as if pulling back against the ball.
- Flex the centre of your back as much as possible when arching it, as if it was being pulled back by someone behind you.

Hints & Tips
- Contract your abdominal muscles when flexing your back to aid the range of the stretch.

spinal lateral flexion

Area Worked: Muscles at the side of your spine and torso
Name of Main Muscle Groups: External Obliques, Quadratus Lumborum, and Latissimus Dorsi

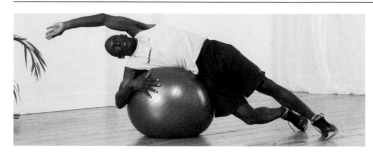

1 Lie sideways onto the Swiss ball. Extend your outside arm above your head, and lower your hand towards the floor. Alternatively, wrap your inside arm around the ball to help your balance.

2 Arch your body over the ball so that you can feel a stretch all the way down your side. Hold this position for 15–20 seconds, and then repeat on your other side.

Technique

- Position yourself so that your side is in the middle of the top of the ball.
- Extend your outside leg, and move your inside leg back a little to aid stability.

Hints & Tips

- Inflating the Swiss Ball to its maximum will create a bigger stretch down your side.

seated pelvic rotations

Areas Worked: Stretch and mobility for the muscles around the lower back and pelvis.
Name of Main Muscle Groups: External Obliques, Internal Obliques

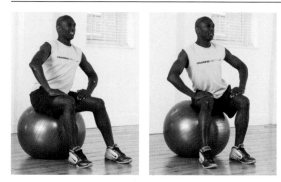

1 Sit on the ball with your feet flat on the floor.

2 Rotate your pelvis, forming large circles to the side, front, side, and back. Repeat this movement for 10 repetitions clockwise, and then counter clockwise.

Technique

- Place yourself directly in the centre of the Swiss Ball.
- Your knees should be bent to 90 degrees.
- Activate and tighten your abdominal muscles.
- Keep your eyes fixed straight ahead so that your neck and back are neutrally aligned.
- Relax your arms and rest your hands on your thighs.
- Keep control throughout the pelvic rotation.

Hints & Tips

- Progressively increase the size of the rotations and circles that you are forming.
- Keeping your feet firmly planted on the floor will help you to control the range of movement.

lumbar rotations

Areas Worked: Stretching and mobility for the soft tissue surrounding the lumbar vertebrae used in rotation of the lower back.

Name of Main Muscle Groups: External Obliques, Erector Spinae

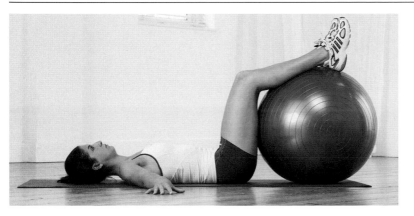

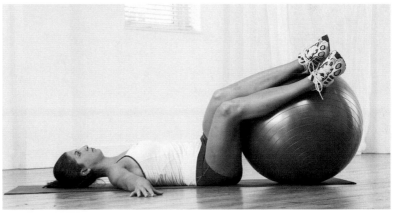

1 Lie on the floor, on your back, with your lower legs resting on top of the Swiss Ball and arms out to the side.

2 Slowly rotate your lower back, rolling the ball and legs over to one side, and pause.

3 Tighten your abdominal muscles and bring your legs back to the starting position.

4 Repeat on the other side, and continue this for 8 to 10 repetitions.

Technique

- Your thighs should be in a vertical position.
- Keep your back flat and in the neutral position.
- Position your arms out to the side to aid stability.
- Move slowly and always through a pain free range.

Hints & Tips

- Relax your abdominal muscle when rolling your legs to the side.
- Focus on your breathing. Breathe out when rotating out to the side and breathe in when returning to the centre.

Lower Body Stretches

lying hamstring stretch

Areas Worked: Back of upper legs
Name of Main Muscle Group: Hamstrings

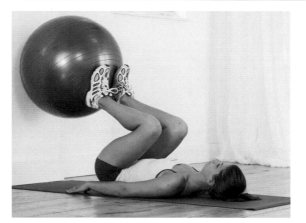

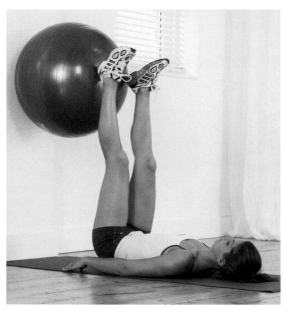

1 Lie on the floor, on your back, with your bottom about a foot away from a wall. Place the Swiss Ball against the wall and hold it there by pushing your feet against it, with your knees bent.

2 Extend your legs so that your heels roll over the ball until your legs become straight.

3 Hold, and then slowly bend your knees rolling your heels back over the ball, and to the starting position.

4 Continue this movement for 8 to 10 repetitions.

Technique

• Maintain your back in a neutral position, not allowing your lower back and pelvis to lift off the floor.
• Move slowly and avoid locking out your knees.
• Position your arms out to the side to aid stability.

Hints & Tips

• Relax your neck and shoulders by keeping your head on the floor.
• Move closer to the wall to increase the stretch. Move further away if the stretch is too intense.
• Breathe out when extending your legs, and breathe in when returning to the starting position.

standing hamstring stretch

Areas Worked: Back of upper legs
Name of Main Muscle Group: Hamstrings

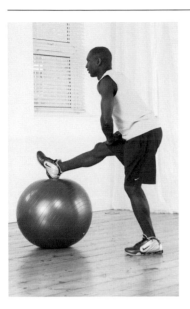

1 Stand on your left leg facing the Swiss Ball. Extend your right leg and place your foot on top of the ball.

2 Gently lean your shoulders forward until you feel a stretch in the back of the right leg. Hold the stretch for 15–20 seconds and then relax, and repeat with your left leg.

Technique

- Stand with your shoulders and hips square on to the Swiss Ball.
- Keep your back neutral and look straight ahead as you shift your weight by leaning your shoulders forward.
- Place your hands on the thigh of the leg that you are stretching but do not push down.

Hints & Tips
- If you are quite inflexible, start with the foot of the leg that you are standing on rotated out at 45 degrees to make it easier.

standing quadriceps stretch

Areas Worked: Front of upper legs
Name of Main Muscle Group: Quadriceps

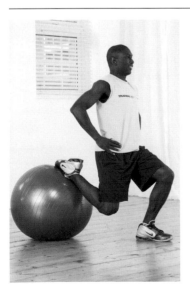

1 Stand on your left leg facing away from the Swiss Ball.

2 Bend your right leg behind you and place your foot on top of the ball.

3 Slowly bend your left leg until you feel a stretch in the front of the right leg.

4 Hold the stretch for 15–20 seconds and then relax, and repeat with your left leg.

Technique

- Keep your back neutral and look straight ahead as you bend the leg that you are standing on.
- The upper part of the leg that you are stretching should be vertical.
- Position yourself so that your standing leg does not bend past 90 degrees.
- Place your hands on your hips.

Hints & Tips
- Activate and tighten your abdominal muscles to help keep yourself balanced and stable.

hip flexor stretch

Areas Worked: Front of hip/thigh
Name of Main Muscle Groups: Psoas and Rectus Femoris

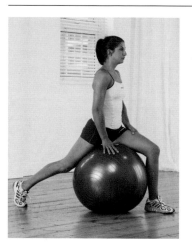

1 Stand over the Swiss Ball, so that your left leg is forward and bent, and your right leg extended back.

2 Bend your left leg, leaning your weight and right thigh into the ball.

3 Hold the stretch for 15–20 seconds and then relax, and repeat with your left leg.

Technique

- Keep your back neutral and look straight ahead.
- Position your body over the centre of the ball with your shoulders and hips facing forward.
- Your front foot should be flat on the floor, but only place the toe of the back foot down.

Hints & Tips

- Lower yourself onto the ball to increase the stretch.
- Place one hand on the ball to steady it.

gluteal stretch

Areas Worked: Muscles in the back of the hip and bottom
Name of Main Muscle Groups: Gluteus Medius and Gluteus Maximus

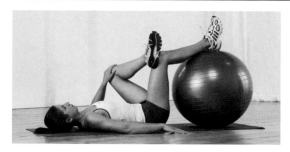

Technique

- Keep your back flat and in the neutral position.
- The thigh of the leg that is on the ball should be vertical.
- Move slowly and always through a pain free range.

1 Lie on the floor, on your back, with the lower part of your right leg resting on top of the Swiss Ball.

2 Rotate your left hip and place the outside of your left ankle over your right knee, which acts as an anchor.

3 Put gentle pressure against the inside of your left knee until you feel a stretch in your left buttock.

4 Hold for 15–20 seconds and repeat on the other side.

Hints & Tips

- Gradually increase the range of the stretch throughout the 15–20 seconds as the muscles lengthen.
- Bringing the knee of the leg that is resting on the ball closer into your body will also increase the stretch.

outer thigh stretch

Areas Worked: Outer thigh and waist
Names of Main Muscle Groups: Gluteus Medius and Quadratus Lumborum

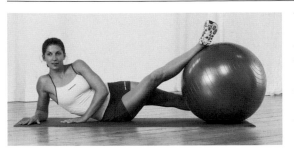

Technique

- Rest your other leg on the floor behind the ball
- Your shoulders and hips should remain in a vertical position throughout the stretch.
- Lift your shoulders slowly as the muscle relaxes and lengthens.
- Keep your hip in contact with the floor during the stretch.

1 Lie on the floor, on your right side.

2 Lift your right leg and rest it on top of the ball.

3 Gently lift your shoulders away from the floor so that you are flexing at the waist.

4 Hold for 15–20 seconds and then repeat on the other side.

Hints & Tips

- Position your hands on the floor to aid stability and hold the stretch.
- Progressively increase the range of the stretch by lifting your shoulders and side away from the floor.

standing inner thigh stretch

Area Worked: Inner thigh
Name of Main Muscle Group: Adductors

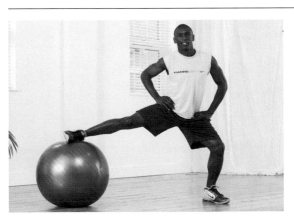

Technique

- Keep your back neutral and look straight ahead as you bend the leg that you are standing on.
- Face your shoulders and hips forward.
- The leg that you are stretching should be completely straight.
- Place your hands on your hips.

1 Stand with the Swiss Ball to your right hand side. Place the inside of your right ankle on the ball, with the leg straight.

2 Slowly bend your left leg, lowering your body, until you feel a stretch in the inner thigh of the right leg.

3 Hold the stretch for 15–20 seconds and then relax, and repeat with your left leg.

Hints & Tips

- Gradually increase the stretch as your inner thigh relaxes.
- Activate and tighten your abdominal muscles to help keep yourself balanced and stable.

Upper Body Stretches

standing chest stretch

Areas Worked: Chest and front of shoulders
Names of Main Muscle Groups: Pectoral and Anterior Deltoid

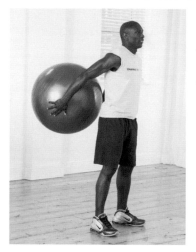

1 Stand up, holding the Swiss Ball behind you with your hands either side.

2 Slowly lift the ball until you can feel the stretch across your chest and front of shoulders.

3 Hold the stretch for 15–20 seconds and then repeat once more.

Technique

- Stand with your feet hip width apart, and knees slightly bent.
- Maintain the neutral position in your back, stopping yourself from leaning forward.
- Keep your head up and eyes fixed straight ahead.
- Your arms should be straight, with the palms of your hands against the ball.

Hints & Tips

- Tighten your abdominals to assist the upright posture.

kneeling chest stretch

Areas Stretched: Chest and front of shoulder
Names of Main Muscle Groups: Pectoral and Anterior Deltoid

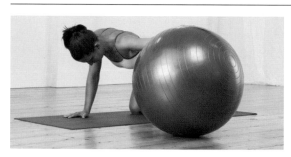

Technique

- Keep your arm stretched out on the ball so that your hand is in line with your shoulder.
- Your other arm and legs should all be positioned vertically.
- Face the floor to keep your neck and back neutrally aligned.
- Your hips and shoulders should be parallel to the floor.

1 Kneel down with the Swiss Ball beside you to your left. Extend your left arm and place your hand on the top of the ball.

2 Slowly lower your left shoulder until you feel the stretch. Hold for 15–20 seconds, and then repeat on the other side using your right arm.

Hints & Tips

- Keep your hips and shoulders parallel to the floor.
- Gradually increase the stretch by lowering your shoulder on the side that you are stretching.

back of shoulder stretch

Areas Worked: Back of shoulder and between the shoulder blades
Names of Main Muscle Groups: Posterior Deltoid and Rhomboids

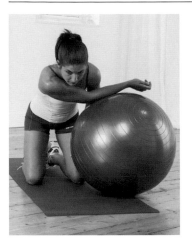

1 Kneel down on the floor with the Swiss Ball in front of you. Place your right arm across your body toward your left shoulder so that it is resting on top of the ball.

2 Lower your shoulders down toward the ball until you can feel a stretch in the back of the right shoulder.

3 Hold this position for 15–20 seconds, and then repeat with your left arm.

Technique

• Rest your forearm and elbow on the ball.
• Keep your shoulders straight and parallel to the floor as you lower them down.

Hints & Tips

• Place your other hand on your thigh to control your weight against the ball.
• Contract your abdominal muscles to hold your back in a neutral position.

single arm lat stretch

Area Worked: Side of upper back
Name of Main Muscle Group: Latissimus Dorsi

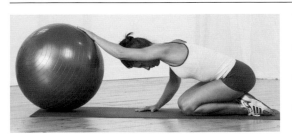

Technique

• Keep your arm stretched out as if pulling back against the ball.
• Face the floor, keeping your neck and back neutrally aligned.
• Your hips and shoulders should be parallel to the floor.

1 Kneel down with the Swiss Ball in front of you.

2 Extend your left arm and place your hand on top of the ball.

3 Slowly sit back onto your heels, and drop your shoulders toward the floor until you feel the stretch.

4 Hold this position for 15–20 seconds, and then repeat with your right arm.

Hints & Tips

• Progressively increase the stretch by lowering your shoulders toward the floor.
• Place your other hand on the floor to help control the height of your shoulders.

combination stretch

Areas Worked: Side of upper back and lower back
Names of Main Muscle Groups: Latissimus Dorsi, External Obliques, and Quadratus Lumborum

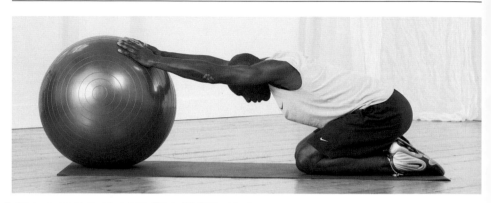

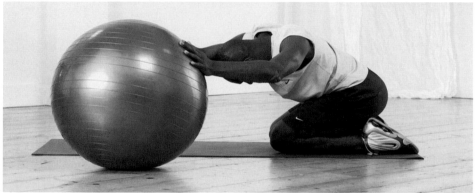

1 Kneel down with the Swiss Ball in front of you. Extend your arms and place your hands on top of the ball. Slowly sit back onto your heels, and drop your shoulders toward the floor until you feel the stretch.

2 Hold this position for 10 seconds, and then roll the ball to your left holding for 10–15 seconds.

3 Finally roll the ball to your right and hold for 10–15 seconds.

Technique

- Keep your arms stretched out as if pulling back against the ball.
- Position your head between your shoulders, facing the floor to keep your neck and back neutrally aligned.
- Your hips and shoulders should be parallel to the floor.
- Roll the ball to each side by walking your hands over the surface of the ball.

Hints & Tips

- Keep your hips and knees facing straight ahead throughout to obtain the best stretch.
- Progressively increase the stretch by lowering your shoulders toward the floor.

shoulder arcs

Area Worked: Mobility of the shoulder
Names of Main Muscle Groups: Anterior/Posterior Deltoid and other deep muscle tissues

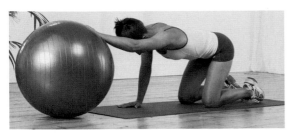

1 Kneel down with the Swiss Ball in front of you. Extend your left arm and place your hand on top of the ball.

2 Slowly roll the ball around, forming an arc at arm's length toward your feet. Hold for a few seconds, and then roll the ball in an arc back to the starting position.

3 Repeat this movement 2 to 3 times, and then do it on the other side using your right arm.

Technique

- Keep your arm stretched out on the ball throughout the movement.
- Your other arm and legs should all be positioned vertically.
- Face the floor to keep your neck and back neutrally aligned.
- Roll the ball to each side by walking your hand over the surface of the ball.

Hints & Tips

- Keep your hips and shoulders parallel to the floor.
- Keeping a light touch with your fingers will help you to roll the ball more smoothly.

upper back rotations

Area Worked: Upper back (vertebrae) mobility
Names of Main Muscle Groups: Latissimus Dorsi, Erector Spinae

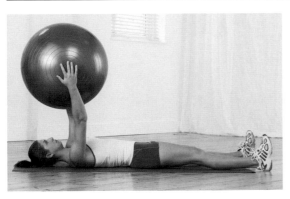

1 Lie on the floor, on your back, with your legs straight. Hold the Swiss Ball up in front of you with your arms straight.

2 Slowly lower the ball to your left until your left hand touches the floor and hold for 3–4 seconds.

3 Return back to the starting position, and repeat on the right hand side. Continue this for 8 repetitions.

Technique

- Hold your back and neck in a neutral position.
- The position of your hands should be directly above your shoulders in the starting position.
- Keep both arms straight as you rotate to each side.
- Make sure that your pelvis stays in contact with the floor throughout the rotations.
- Move slowly and always through a pain free range.

Hints & Tips

- Keep your eyes looking straight up to maintain a neutral neck position.
- Aim to get the arm on the side you are rotating flat on the floor for a full range movement.
- Focus on your breathing. Breathe out when rotating out to the side and breathe in when returning to the center.

Upper Body Exercises
Strength and Tone
Beginner–Intermediate

chest press

Areas Worked: Chest, front of shoulder, back of upper arm, and the core
Names of Main Muscle Groups: Pectorals, Anterior Deltoid, and Triceps

1 Lie on your back on top of the ball in the reverse bridge position, with your knees bent at 90 degrees. Take hold of a dumbbell in each hand with an over-hand grip. Bend your elbows to 90 degrees and position them out level with your shoulders.

2 Extend both arms up, pushing the weights away, until they are straight. Pause and then slowly bend your arms allowing them to return to the start position.

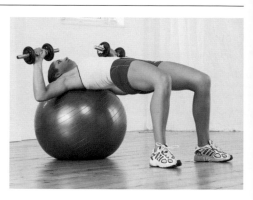

Technique

- The ball should be positioned so that it sits directly between your shoulder blades.
- Place your feet shoulder width apart.
- Activate and tighten your abdominal muscles to help maintain a neutral alignment.
- Be careful not to let your pelvis drop and move out of alignment. You should form a straight line from your shoulders through to your knees.
- Ensure that your forearms maintain a vertical position throughout the movement.
- Stop at the bottom of the movement when you feel a stretch across your chest and shoulders.

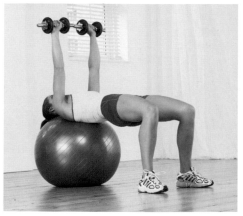

Hints & Tips

- Your foot position has a huge impact on how difficult the exercise is with regards to stability. The closer your feet are together the less stable you will be. Start by placing them shoulder width apart; as you improve, gradually bring them closer together.
- Breathe out as you extend your arms and push the weights up, breathe in as you return.

alternate arm chest press

Areas Worked: Chest, front of shoulder, and back of upper arm as a main focus. The alternate arm version allows you to work one arm at a time while increasing the instability and activating the muscles of the core.
Names of Main Muscle Groups: Pectorals, Anterior Deltoid, and Triceps

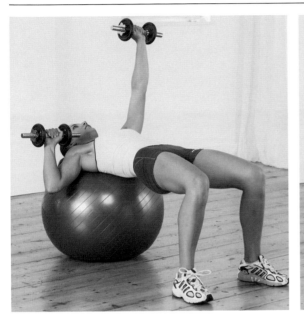 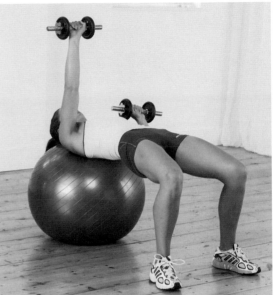

1　Lie on your back on top of the ball in the reverse bridge position, with your knees bent at 90 degrees. Take hold of a dumbbell in each hand with an over-hand grip. Bend your elbows to 90 degrees and position them out level with your shoulders.

2　Extend one arm up, pushing the weight away, until it is straight. Pause and then slowly bend your arm allowing it to return to the start position.

3　Repeat this action with your other arm, continuing this alternate arm action for the desired number of repetitions.

Technique

- Position the ball so that it sits directly between your shoulder blades.
- Place your feet shoulder width apart.
- Activate and tighten your abdominal muscles to help maintain a neutral alignment.
- Be careful not to let your pelvis drop and move out of alignment.
- Ensure that your forearms maintain a vertical position throughout each movement and while static.
- Stop at the bottom of the movement when you feel a stretch across your chest and shoulder.
- While extending one arm, keep the other bent and static, then extend once the first arm has reached the bottom of its movement.

Hints & Tips

- Your foot position has a huge impact on how difficult the exercise is with regards to stability. The closer your feet are together the less stable you will be. Start by placing them shoulder width apart; as you improve, gradually bring them closer together.
- Breathe out as you extend your arms and push the weights up. Breathe in as you return.

pectoral fly

Areas Worked: Chest, front of shoulder, and the core
Names of Main Muscle Groups: Pectorals and Anterior Deltoid

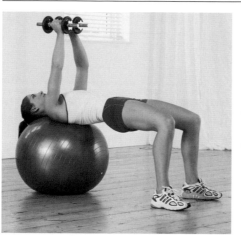

1 Lie on your back on top of the ball in the reverse bridge position with your knees bent at 90 degrees. Take hold of a dumbbell in each hand with a palms-in grip. Start with both arms extended and hands above your shoulders.

2 Slowly lower your arms out to the side in an arc, until you feel a stretch across your chest.

3 Pause and then raise your arms back up to the starting position following the same arc.

Technique

- The ball should be positioned so that it sits directly between your shoulder blades.
- Place your feet shoulder width apart.
- Activate and tighten your abdominal muscles to help maintain a neutral alignment.
- Be careful not to let your pelvis drop and move out of alignment. You should form a straight line from your shoulders through to your knees.
- Keep a slight bend in your elbows and fix them in that position throughout the exercise.
- As you lower your arm, keep your hand in line with your shoulder.
- Stop at the bottom of the movement when you feel a stretch across your chest.

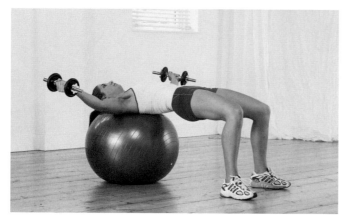

Hints & Tips

- Keep your eyes fixed on a point on the ceiling.
- Your foot position will impact your stability. The closer your feet are together the less stable you will be. Start by placing them shoulder width apart.
- Breathe out as you arc your arms up, breathe in as you lower your arms down.

Strength and Tone
Advanced

incline dumbbell chest press

Areas Worked: Upper Chest, front of shoulders, and back of upper arms
Names of Main Muscle Groups: Upper Pectorals, Anterior Deltoid, and Triceps

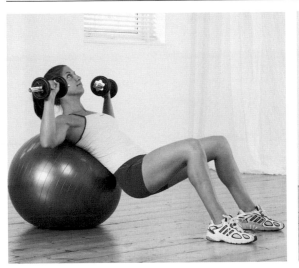 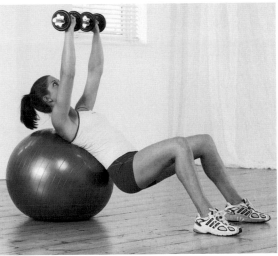

1 Lie with your back against the Swiss Ball, with your knees bent at 90 degrees. Drop your hips down until your torso is at a 45-degree angle. Take hold of a dumbbell in each hand with an over-hand grip. Bend your elbows to 90 degrees and position them out level with your shoulders.

2 Extend both arms up, pushing the weights away, until they are straight.

3 Pause and then slowly bend your arms, allowing them to return to the start position.

Technique

- Position yourself so that your back is arched against the ball.
- Place your feet shoulder width apart.
- Activate and tighten your abdominal muscles to help maintain control of your midsection.
- Ensure that your forearms maintain a vertical position throughout the movement.
- Stop at the bottom of the movement when you feel a stretch across your chest and shoulders.

Hints & Tips

- The closer your feet are together the less stable you will be.
- Although your body is at a 45-degree angle, your arms should still extend vertically.
- Breathe out as you extend your arms and push the weights up, breathe in as you return.

single arm chest press

Areas Worked: Chest, front of shoulder, back of upper arm, and the core muscle groups
Names of Main Muscle Groups: Pectorals, Anterior Deltoid, and Triceps

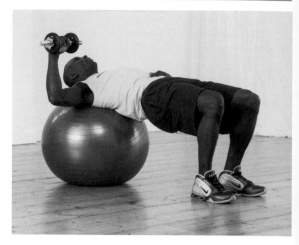

1 Lie on your back on top of the ball in the reverse bridge position, with your knees bent at 90 degrees. Take hold of a dumbbell in one hand. Bend your elbow to 90 degrees and position it out level with your shoulders.

2 Extend your arm up, pushing the weight away, until it is straight.

3 Pause and then slowly bend your arm allowing it to return to the start position.

4 Continue for the desired number of repetitions and then repeat this action using your other arm.

Technique

- Position yourself on the ball so that it sits directly between your shoulder blades
- Place your feet hip width apart.
- Activate and tighten your abdominal muscles to help maintain a neutral alignment.
- Be careful not to let your pelvis drop and move out of alignment.
- Ensure that your forearm maintains a vertical position throughout each movement and while static.
- Rest your other hand on your stomach.
- Stop at the bottom of the movement when you feel a stretch across your chest and shoulder.

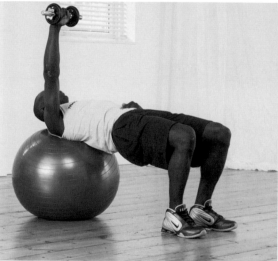

Hints & Tips

- As always, choose your foot position carefully as it will impact the difficulty of the exercise.
- Remember, the closer your feet are together the less stable you will be.
- Maintain control of the movement to feel all the areas working.
- Breathe out as you extend your arm and push the weight up. Breathe in as you return.

single arm pectoral fly

Areas Worked: Chest, front of shoulder, and particularly the core
Names of Main Muscle Groups: Pectorals and Anterior Deltoid

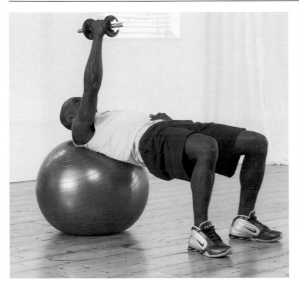 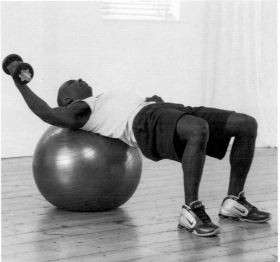

1 Lie on your back on top of the ball in the reverse bridge position with your knees bent at 90 degrees. Take hold of a dumbbell in one hand with a palm-in grip. Start with one arm extended and your other arm relaxed, with your hand resting on your stomach.

2 Slowly lower your arm out to the side in an arc, until you feel a stretch across your chest.

3 Pause and then raise your arm back up to the starting position, following the same arc.

Technique

- The ball should be positioned so that it sits directly between your shoulder blades.
- Place your feet shoulder width apart.
- Maintain a neutral alignment by activating and tightening your abdominal muscles.
- You should hold a straight line from your shoulders through to your knees.
- Keep a slight bend in your elbow and fix it in that position throughout the exercise.
- Stop at the bottom of the movement when you feel a stretch across your chest.

Hints & Tips

- This exercise demands you to stabilize yourself more than the others chest exercises, so start by placing your feet shoulder width apart and gradually move them closer as you improve.
- Keep your eyes fixed on a point on the ceiling.
- Breathe out as you raise your arm, breathe in as you lower your arm.

Balance and Stability
Beginner–Intermediate

press ups, kneeling on the floor

Areas Worked: Chest, front of shoulders, back of upper arms, and core
Names of Main Muscle Groups: Pectorals, Anterior Deltoid, and Triceps

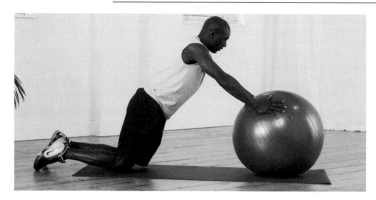

1 Kneel on the floor leaning forward, with your arms extended and hands resting on top of the ball.

2 Bend your arms bringing your chest toward the ball until your elbows reach 90 degrees.

3 Pause, and then extend your arms pushing your chest away from the ball and returning to the start position.

Technique

- Activate and tighten your abdominal muscles to help maintain a neutral back position.
- Pivot on your knees as you lower your upper body toward the ball.
- Your elbows should move out to the side as you bend your arms.
- Stop at the bottom of the movement when you feel a stretch across your chest and shoulders.

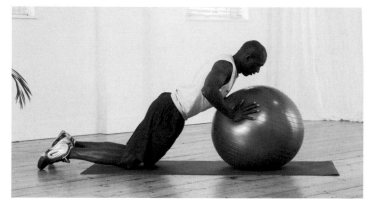

Hints & Tips
- Position your hands wide apart on the ball to assist stability.
- Breathe in as you bend your arms and lower yourself down, breathe out as you extend your arms.

press ups, toes on the floor

Areas Worked: Chest, front of shoulders, back of upper arms, and core
Names of Main Muscle Groups: Pectorals, Anterior Deltoid, Triceps, and Transversus Abdominus

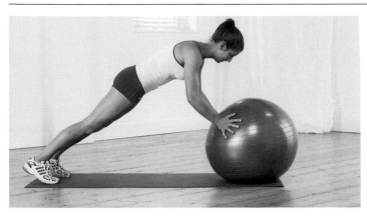

1 Position yourself on your toes with your arms extended and hands resting on top of the ball.

2 Bend your arms bringing your chest toward the ball until your elbows reach 90 degrees.

3 Pause, and then extend your arms pushing your chest away from the ball and returning to the start position.

Technique

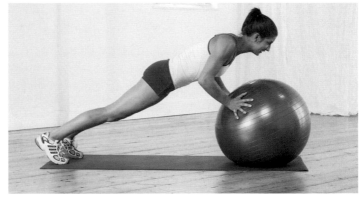

- Activate and tighten your core muscles to maintain a neutral position with a straight line running from your shoulders to your ankles.
- Pivot on your toes as you lower your upper body toward the ball.
- Your elbows should move out to the side as you bend your arms.
- Stop at the bottom of the movement when you feel a stretch across your chest and shoulders.

Hints & Tips

- Position your hands wide apart on the ball to assist stability.
- Your foot position will also affect the difficulty of the exercise (closer is harder).
- Breathe in as you bend your arms and lower yourself down. Breathe out as you extend your arms.

Balance and Stability
Advanced

press ups, toes on the ball

Areas Worked: Chest, front of shoulders, back of upper arms, and core
Names of Main Muscle Groups: Upper Pectorals, Anterior Deltoid, Triceps, and Transversus Abdominus

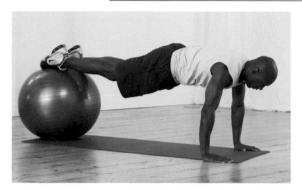

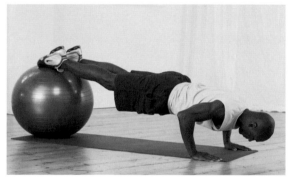

1 Position yourself on your hands with arms extended and toes resting on top of the ball.

2 Bend your arms, bringing your chest toward the floor until elbows reach 90 degrees.

3 Pause, and then extend your arms pushing your chest away from the floor and returning to the start position.

Technique

- Position your hands on the floor so that they are directly below your shoulders.
- Activate and tighten your core muscles to maintain a neutral position with a straight line running from your shoulders to your ankles.
- Make sure that your back doesn't arch during the exercise.
- Face the floor throughout the movement to keep your neck neutrally aligned.
- Your elbows should move out to the side as you bend your arms.
- Avoid locking your elbows when your arms are straight.

Hints & Tips

- Your hand position will greatly affect the difficulty of the exercise, with a close position being harder.
- Focus on keeping your body from your neck to your ankles in a straight line. Imagine that you are a ridged plank.
- Breathe in as you bend your arms and lower yourself down. Breathe out as you extend your arms.

Back Exercises
Strength and Tone
Beginner–Intermediate

mid row

Areas Worked: Upper back, between shoulder blades, back of shoulders, and front of upper arms
Names of Main Muscle Groups: Lower Trapezius, Rhomboids, Posterior Deltoid, and Biceps

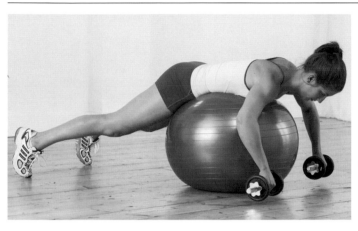

1 Position yourself face down on the Swiss Ball with your legs stretched out and your toes on the floor.

2 Start with your upper arms out to the side and extended down toward the floor, taking hold of the weights with an overhand grip.

3 Lift your elbows up past shoulder level, bending your arms.

4 Pause, and then extend your arms returning the weights back toward the floor.

Technique

- Your elbows should move out to the side at a 90 degree angle as you flex your arms.
- Stop at the bottom of the movement, making sure that the weights don't touch the floor.
- Ensure that your forearms are vertically positioned throughout the exercise.
- Keep your torso still during the movement.
- Make sure that your shoulders do not lift away from the ball as you raise your elbows.

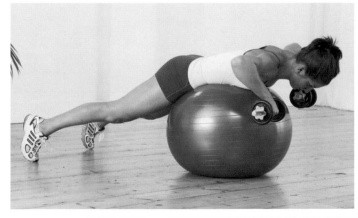

Hints & Tips

- Hold your legs straight to maintain the correct position on the ball.
- Squeeze your shoulder blades together at the top of the movement to work the Rhomboids through a full range.
- Your foot position will also affect the difficulty of the exercise (closer is harder).
- Breathe out as you flex your arms and lift your elbows, breathe in as you extend your arms back down.

kneeling back extension

Area Worked: Length of back
Name of Main Muscle Group: Erector Spinae

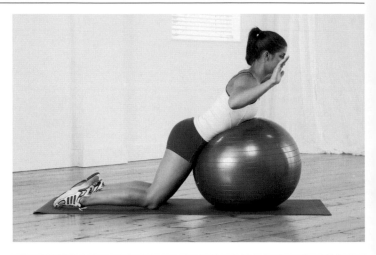

1 Kneel on the floor, and lean onto the Swiss Ball, resting all your weight down.

2 Extend your back, lifting your chest away from the ball.

3 Pause, and then lower your chest back down to the ball and start position.

Technique

- When kneeling, your thighs should be at approximately a 45-degree angle from knee to hip.
- Hold your arms out at a 90-degree angle to your body with your elbows bent.
- Position your head so that you are facing the floor just ahead of you throughout the exercise.

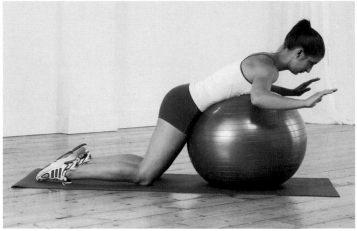

Hints & Tips

- Squeeze your shoulders blades together and pull your arms back as you extend your back to feel the length of your back working.
- Push your hips into the ball as you lift your chest away.
- Breathe out as you extend your back, breathe in as you lower your chest back down.

back extension with toes on floor

Area Worked: Length of back
Name of Main Muscle Group: Erector Spinae

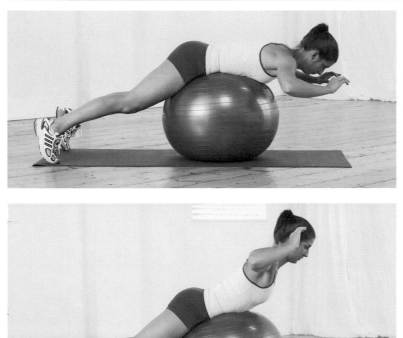

1 Lie on the Swiss Ball face down, so that your navel is on the center of the ball, and your legs are extended.

2 Extend your back by lifting your chest away from the ball.

3 Pause, and then lower your chest back down to the ball and start position.

Technique

- Keep your legs extended straight behind you, with your toes on the floor.
- Hold your arms out at a 90-degree angle to your body with your elbows bent.
- Position your head so that you are facing the floor just ahead of you throughout the exercise.

Hints & Tips

- Squeeze your shoulder blades together and pull your arms back as you extend your back to feel the length of your back working.
- Push your hips into the ball as you lift your chest away.
- Find the best position for your toes on the floor for stability and grip.
- Breathe out as you extend your back, breathe in as you lower your chest back down.

Strength and Tone
Advanced

single arm mid row

Areas Worked: Upper back, between shoulder blades, back of shoulder and front of upper arm
Names of Main Muscle Groups: Lower Trapezius, Rhomboids, Posterior Deltoid, and Biceps

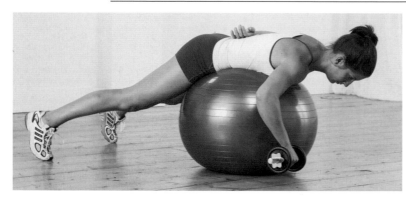

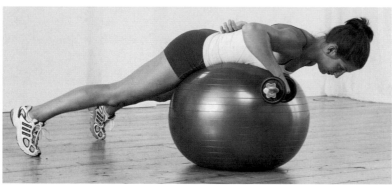

1 Lie face down on the Swiss Ball, with your legs stretched out and your toes on the floor.

2 Start with one upper arm out to the side and extended down toward the floor, holding the weight in an over-hand grip.

3 Lift your elbow up past shoulder level, bending your arm.

4 Pause, and then extend your arm returning the weight back toward the floor.

5 Repeat with your other arm.

Technique

- Position your elbow out to the side at a 90-degree angle as you flex your arm.
- Stop at the bottom of the movement, making sure that the weight doesn't touch the floor.
- Ensure that your forearm is vertically positioned throughout the exercise.
- Place your other arm behind your back with the palm of your hand facing upward.
- Keep your torso still during the movement.
- Stop your shoulders from lifting away from the ball as you raise your elbows.

Hints & Tips

- Start with a wide foot placement, and move them closer as you develop your strengths and balance.
- Hold your legs straight to maintain the correct position on the ball.
- Breathe out as you flex your arm and lift your elbow, breathe in as you extend your arm back down.

bent over single arm row

Areas Worked: Upper back, between shoulder blades, back of shoulder, and front of upper arm
Names of Main Muscle Groups: Lower Trapezius, Rhomboids, Posterior Deltoid, and Biceps

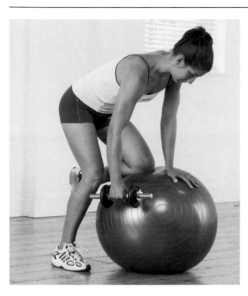
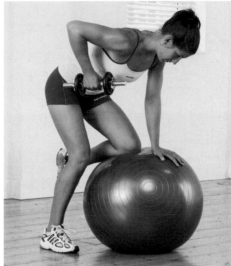

1 Position yourself with your left knee and left hand on the Swiss Ball, and your right foot flat on the floor. Take hold of a weight with your right hand using a palms-in grip. Start with your right arm extended down toward the floor.

2 Flex your arm lifting your elbow up and past shoulder level. Pause, and then extend your arm returning the weight back toward the floor.

3 Repeat with your left arm, placing your right hand and knee on the ball.

Technique

- Neutrally align your back and neck, fixing them in that position.
- Start with your arm straight and vertical.
- Position your elbow tight to your body as you bring the weight up, with your forearm vertical.
- Hold your shoulders and hips parallel to the floor throughout the exercise.
- Keep your torso still during the movement.

Hints & Tips

- Aim to lift your elbow past the line of your shoulders for a full range movement.
- Control your position and balance with the leg that is in contact with the floor.
- Breathe out as you flex your arm and lift your elbow, breathe in as you extend your arm back down.

49

weighted back extension

Area Worked: Length of back
Name of Main Muscle Group: Erector Spinae

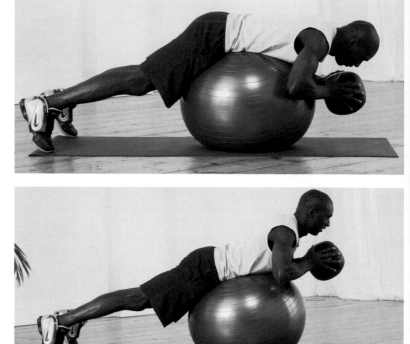

1 Lie face down on the Swiss Ball with your legs extended. Take hold of the medicine ball with both hands, and position it just below your chin.

2 Extend your back, lifting your chest away from the ball.

3 Pause, and then lower your chest back down to the ball and start position.

Technique

- Hold your arms and ball in the same position with your elbows pointing out throughout the movement.
- Keep your legs extended straight behind you with your toes on the floor.
- Position your head so that you are facing the floor.

Hints & Tips

- Push your hips into the ball as you lift your chest away.
- Find the best position for your toes on the floor for stability and grip.
- To make the exercise harder you can extend your arms moving the ball further away from your body.
- Breathe out as you extend your back, breathe in as you lower your chest back down.

Balance and Stability
Beginner–Intermediate

mid row, leg extended

Areas Worked: Upper back, between shoulder blades, back of shoulders, front of upper arms, and core for stability
Names of Main Muscle Groups: Lower Trapezius, Rhomboids, Posterior Deltoid, and Biceps

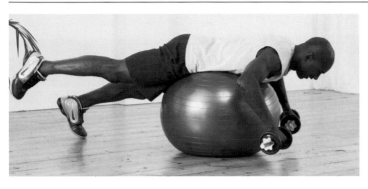

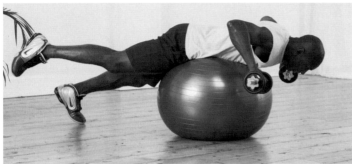

1 Lie face down on the Swiss Ball with your right leg elevated off the floor and the toes of your left leg on the floor. Start with your upper arms out to the side and extended down toward the floor, holding the weights with an over-hand grip.

2 Lift your elbows up past shoulder level, bending your arms. Pause, and then extend your arms, returning the weights back toward the floor

3 Repeat, elevating your left leg.

Technique

• Hold your leg extended and foot off the floor for the duration of the exercise.
• Focus on control and keeping balanced as you lift the weights.
• Position your elbows out to the side at a 90-degree angle as you flex your arms.
• Stop at the bottom of the movement, making sure that the weights don't touch the floor.
• Ensure that your forearms are vertically positioned throughout the exercise.
• Keep your torso still during the movement.
• Make sure that your shoulders do not lift away from the ball as you raise your elbows.

Hints & Tips

• Activate your core muscles to become stable on the ball with only the one foot in contact with the floor.
• Squeeze your shoulder blades together at the top of the movement.
• Breathe out as you flex your arms and lift your elbows, breathe in as you extend your arms back down.

alternate arm and leg back extensions

Area Worked: Length of back
Name of Main Muscle Group: Erector Spinae

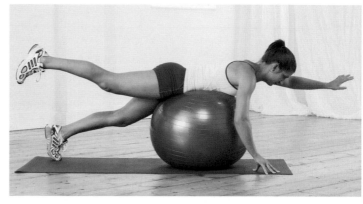

1 Lie on the Swiss Ball face down with your arms and legs extended. Extend your back, lifting your left arm and right leg off the floor.

2 Hold for 3 seconds, and then lower your arm and leg back to the floor.

3 Repeat the exercise with your right arm and left leg.

Technique

- Place the opposite hand and toe on the floor to those that are elevated.
- Keep your arms and legs straight both when lifting and when static.
- Position your head so that you are facing the floor.

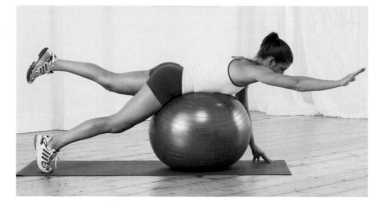

Hints & Tips

- Keep your body weight directly in the center of the ball to aid stability.
- To make the exercise harder you can hold your arm and leg up for a longer period of time.
- Breathe out as you lift your arm and leg, breathe in as you lower them back down.

Balance and Stability
Advanced

latissimus ball roll

Areas Worked: Side of back, back of shoulders, and core
Name of Main Muscle Groups: Latissimus Dorsi, Posterior Deltoid, Rectus Abdominus, and Transversus Abdominus

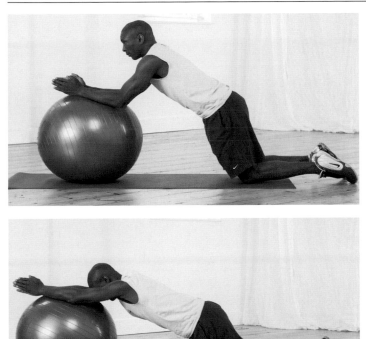

1 Kneel on the floor, leaning forward with your arms bent to 90 degrees, and rest your forearms on top of the Swiss Ball.

2 Slowly extend your arms forward, lowering your shoulders as you roll the ball away.

3 Hold the position for a few seconds, and then pull your elbows back, rolling the ball back and raising your shoulders, until you reach the start position.

Technique

- Activate and tighten your abdominal muscles to help maintain a neutral back position.
- Pivot on your knees as you lower and raise your shoulders, fixing your hips in position.
- Your elbows should end up resting on top of the ball when your arms are fully extended.
- Stop at the bottom of the movement when you feel a stretch under your shoulders and down the side of your upper back.

Hints & Tips

- To find your starting point, slowly roll forward until you feel your abdominals beginning to work.
- Keep your pelvis tilted back slightly throughout the movement to prevent stress on your lower back.
- Breathe in as you extend your arms and lower yourself down, breathe out as you pull your arms back.

Shoulder Exercises
Strength and Tone
Beginner–Intermediate

seated shoulder press

Areas Worked: Front of shoulders and back of upper arms
Names of Main Muscle Groups: Anterior Deltoid and Triceps

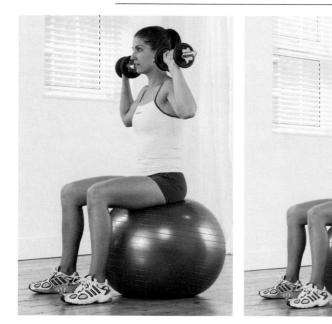

1 Sit on the ball with your feet flat on the floor. Take hold of a weight in both hands with an over-hand grip, positioning them just above shoulder level.

2 Extend your arms, pushing the weights above your head.

3 Pause, and then flex your arms, lowering the weights back down to the start position.

Technique

- Place yourself directly in the center of the Swiss Ball.
- Knees should be bent to 90 degrees.
- Activate and tighten your abdominal muscles.
- Keep your eyes fixed straight ahead so that your neck and back are neutrally aligned.
- Start with your elbows pointed out to the side, keeping your forearms vertical.
- Extend your arms straight up so that they are vertical when fully extended.

Hints & Tips

- Keeping your feet firmly planted on the floor will help you balance.
- Activate your abdominals to maintain stability as you are lifting the weights above your head.
- Breathe out as you extend your arms. Breathe in as you lower them down.

seated lateral raise

Area Worked: Top of shoulders
Names of Main Muscle Groups: Medial Deltoid and Upper Trapezius

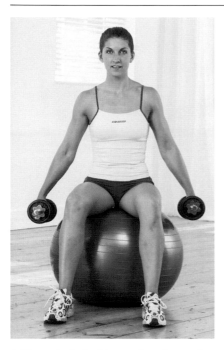 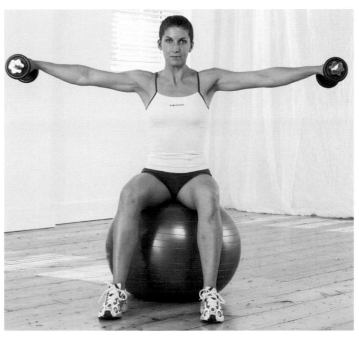

1 Sit on the ball with your feet flat on the floor. Take hold of a weight in both hands with an over-hand grip, positioning them down by your side

2 Lift your arms up and out to the side until the weights are at shoulder height.

3 Pause, and then lower your arms, returning the weights back down to the start position.

Technique

- Place yourself on the center of the Swiss Ball.
- Your knees should be bent to 90 degrees.
- Activate and tighten your abdominal muscles.
- Keep your eyes fixed straight ahead so that your neck and back are neutrally aligned.
- Ensure that your arms stay straight throughout the movement.

Hints & Tips

- Keep your feet firmly planted on the floor to help you balance on the ball.
- Activate your abdominals to maintain stability and a neutral posture with your shoulders back and chest out.
- Breathe out as you lift your arms. Breathe in as you lower them down.

seated front raise

Area Worked: Front of shoulders
Name of Main Muscle Group: Anterior Deltoid

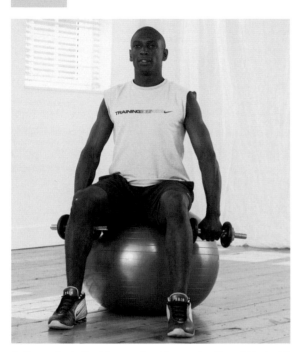

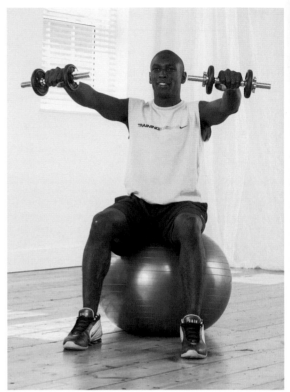

1 Sit on the ball with your feet flat on the floor. Take hold of a weight in both hands with an over-hand grip, positioning them down by your side.

2 Lift your arms forward and up until the weights are at shoulder height.

3 Pause, and then lower your arms, returning the weights back down to the start position.

Technique

- Position yourself on the center of the Swiss Ball.
- Your knees should be bent to 90 degrees.
- Activate and tighten your abdominal muscles.
- Keep your eyes fixed straight ahead so that your neck and back are neutrally aligned.
- Ensure that your arms stay straight throughout the movement.

Hints & Tips

- Keep your feet firmly planted on the floor to help you balance on the ball.
- Activate your abdominals to maintain stability and a neutral posture with your shoulders back and chest out.
- Breathe out as you lift your arms. Breathe in as you lower them down.

prone lateral raise

Area Worked: Back of shoulder
Name of Main Muscle Group: Posterior Deltoid

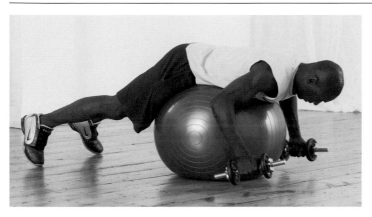

1 Lie face down on the Swiss Ball, with your legs stretched out and toes on the floor. Take hold of the weights with a palms-in grip. Start with your arms out to the side and extended down toward the floor with a slight bend in the elbow.

2 Lift your elbows up past shoulder level, keeping your arms in a fixed position.

3 Pause, and then lower your arms, returning the weights back toward the floor.

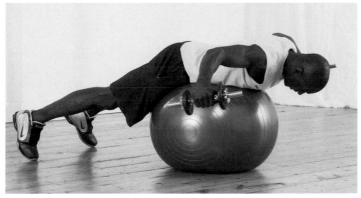

Technique

- Hold your arms in the slightly bent position throughout the exercise.
- Lift your elbows as high as you can, ensuring that they both reach the same height.
- Your hands should remain in line with your shoulders at all times.
- Stop at the bottom of the movement, making sure that the weights don't touch the floor.
- Keep your torso still during the movement.
- Make sure that your shoulders do not lift away from the ball as you raise your arms out to the side.

Hints & Tips

- Hold your legs straight to maintain the correct position on the ball.
- Squeeze your shoulder blades together at the top to encourage a full range of movement.
- Breathe out as you lift your arms out, breathe in as you lower your arms back down.

57

windmills

Areas Worked: Deep muscles stabilizing the shoulder girdle
Name of Main Muscle Group: Rotator Cuff

1 Lie face down on the Swiss Ball with your legs straight and toes on the floor.

2 Start with your upper arms at right angles to your body, and your elbows bent to a 90-degree angle.

3 Using an over-hand grip, internally rotate your left shoulder, moving the weight toward your hip, and externally rotate your right shoulder, lifting the weight up toward head level.

4 Pause, and then swap positions, internally rotating your right shoulder toward your hip and externally rotating your left shoulder toward head level.

Technique

- Your upper arms should stay fixed at right angles to your body throughout the movement.
- Synchronize the movements so that both shoulders are being rotated simultaneously.
- Keep your torso still during the movement.

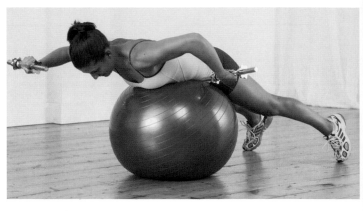

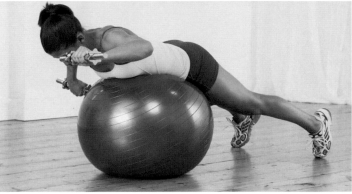

Hints & Tips

- Hold your legs straight to maintain the correct position on the ball.
- Imagine that you have got a broom handle running across the back of your shoulders to either elbow, fixing your upper arms in position. Squeezing your shoulder blades together will also help you.
- Keep checking your elbows to ensure that they are not raising or dropping as you rotate your shoulders.
- Breathe out as you rotate your shoulders and lift your hands.

external shoulder rotation

Areas Worked: Deep muscles stabilizing the shoulder girdle
Name of Main Muscle Group: Rotator Cuff

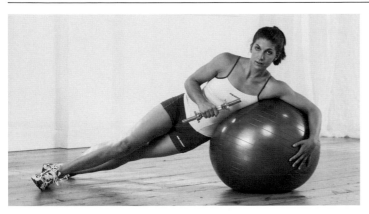

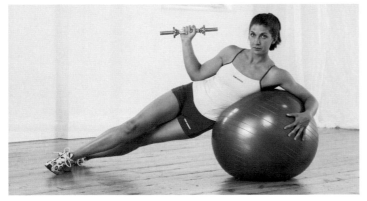

1 Lie on your right hand side against the Swiss Ball, legs extended, and feet on the floor. Bend flex your arm to a 90-degree angle, and rest your elbow on your hip with your hand dropped down toward the floor.

2 Externally rotate your shoulder, raising your hand and pivoting your elbow on your hip.

3 Pause, and slowly lower your hand, returning back to the start position.

Technique

- Keep your elbow positioned on your hip as you externally rotate your shoulder.
- Stop at the bottom of the movement before your forearm makes contact with your stomach.
- Activate and tighten your abdominal muscles to help maintain a neutral back position.

Hints & Tips

- Stabilize your shoulders and hip in a vertical position so that you can focus on the external rotation of the shoulder.
- Stagger the placement of your feet, one in front of the other, to keep yourself balanced.
- Breathe out as you rotate your shoulder and raise the weight up. Breathe in as you lower the weight back down.

Strength and Tone
Advanced

single arm seated lateral raise

Area Worked: Top of shoulder
Names of Main Muscle Groups: Medial Deltoid and Upper Trapezius

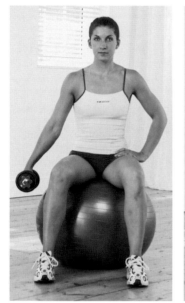 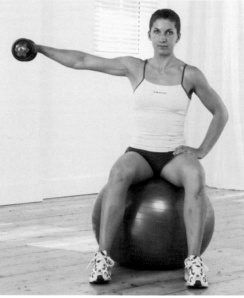

1 Sit on the ball with your feet flat on the floor. Take hold of a weight in one hand with an overhand grip, positioning it down by your side.

2 Lift your arm up and out to the side until the weight is at shoulder height.

3 Pause, and then lower your arm returning the weight back down to the start position.

4 Repeat the exercise using your other arm.

Technique

- Place yourself on the center of the Swiss Ball.
- Your knees should be bent to 90 degrees .
- Activate and tighten your abdominal muscles.
- Avoid leaning your body away from the weight as you lift it.
- Keep your eyes fixed straight ahead so that your neck and back are neutrally aligned.
- Ensure that your arm stays straight throughout the movement.
- Rest your other hand on your hip.

Hints & Tips

- Keep your feet firmly planted on the floor to help you balance on the ball.
- Activate your abdominals to maintain stability and a neutral posture, with your shoulders back and chest out.
- Breathe out as you lift your arm. Breathe in as you lower it back down.

single arm prone lateral raise

Area Worked: Back of shoulder
Name of Main Muscle Group: Posterior Deltoid

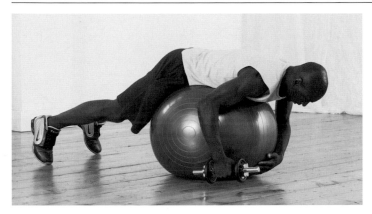

1 Lie face down on the Swiss Ball with your legs stretched out and toes on the floor. Take hold of the weight in one hand with a palms-in grip. Start with your arm out to the side and extended down toward the floor with a slight bend in the elbow.

2 Lift your elbow up past shoulder level, keeping your arm fixed in position.

3 Pause, and then lower your arm, returning the weight back toward the floor.

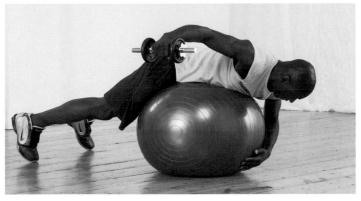

Technique

- Hold your arm in the slightly bent position throughout the exercise.
- Lift your elbow as high as you can toward shoulder height.
- The hand of your weighted arm should remain in line with your shoulder at all times.
- Stop at the bottom of the movement, making sure that the weight doesn't touch the floor.
- Keep your torso still during the movement.
- Make sure that your shoulder does not lift away from the ball as you raise your arm out to the side.

Hints & Tips

- Hold your legs straight to maintain the correct position on the ball.
- Position your hand around the front of the ball for support.
- Squeeze your shoulder blades together at the top to encourage a full range of movement.
- Breathe out as you lift your arm out, breathe in as you lower your arm back down.

61

Balance and Stability
Beginner–Intermediate

seated shoulder press, leg extended

Areas Worked: Front of shoulders, back of upper arms, and core
Names of Main Muscle Groups: Anterior Deltoid and Triceps

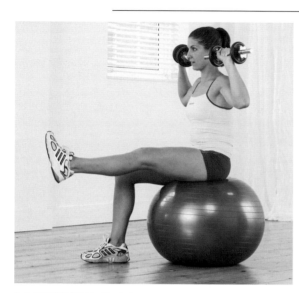

1 Sit on the ball with your right foot flat on the floor. Take hold of a weight in both hands with an over-hand grip, positioning them just above shoulder level. Lift and extend your left leg so that it is horizontal.

2 Extend your arms, pushing the weights above your head.

3 Pause, and then flex your arms, lowering the weights back down to the start position.

4 Repeat, extending your right leg off the floor.

Technique

- Place yourself directly in the center of the Swiss Ball.
- Extend one leg completely straight and hold it in position for the duration of the exercise.
- The knee of the stabilizing leg should be bent to 90 degrees with your foot flat on the floor.
- Activate and tighten your abdominal muscles.
- Keep your eyes fixed straight ahead so that your neck and back are neutrally aligned.
- Start with your elbows pointed out to the side, keeping your forearms vertical.
- Extend your arms straight up so that they are vertical when fully extended.

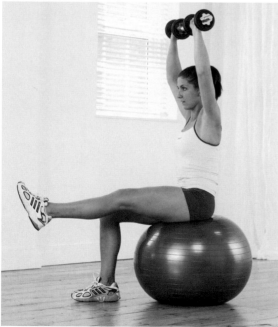

Hints & Tips

- Activate your abdominals to maintain stability and a neutral posture as you are lifting the weights above your head.
- Breathe out as you extend your arms. Breathe in as you lower them down.

alternate arm shoulder press, leg extended

Areas Worked: Front of shoulders, back of upper arms, and core
Names of Main Muscle Groups: Anterior Deltoid and Triceps

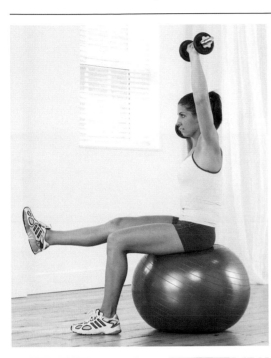

1 Sit on the ball with your left foot flat on the floor. Take hold of a weight in both hands, positioning them just above shoulder level. Lift and extend your right leg so that it is horizontal.

2 Extend your left arm, pushing the weight above your head.

3 Pause, and then flex your arm, lowering the weight back down to the starting position.

4 Repeat, extending your right arm above your head.

Technique

- Place yourself directly on the center of the Swiss Ball.
- Extend one leg completely straight and hold it in position for the duration of the exercise.
- The knee of the stabilizing leg should be bent to 90 degrees with your foot flat on the floor.
- Activate and tighten your abdominal muscles.
- Keep your eyes fixed straight ahead so that your neck and back are neutrally aligned.
- Start with your elbows pointed out to the side, keeping your forearms vertical.
- Extend your arm straight up so that it is vertical when fully extended.
- Hold your other arm just above shoulder height until your active arm returns to the start position.

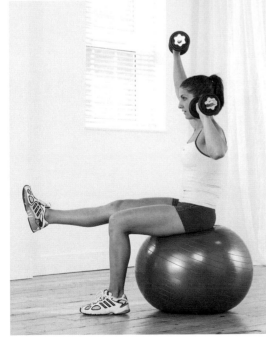

Hints & Tips

- Activate your abdominals to maintain stability and a neutral posture as you are lifting the weights above your head.
- Breathe out as you extend your arms. Breathe in as you lower them down.

lateral raise, leg extended

Areas Worked: Top of shoulders and core
Names of Main Muscle Groups: Medial Deltoid and Upper Trapezius

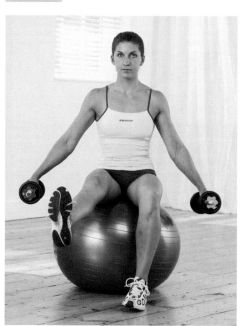
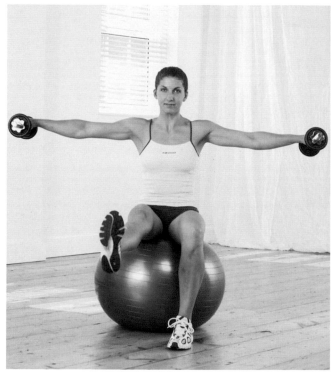

1 Sit on the ball with your left foot flat on the floor. Take hold of a weight in both hands with an over-hand grip, positioning them down by your side.

2 Lift and extend your right leg so that it is horizontal.

3 Raise your arms up and out to the side until the weights are at shoulder height.

4 Pause, and then lower your arms, returning the weights back down to the starting position.

5 Repeat, extending your left leg off the floor.

Technique

- Place yourself directly in the center of the Swiss Ball.
- Extend one leg completely straight and hold it in position for the duration of the exercise.
- The knee of the stabilizing leg should be bent to 90 degrees with one foot flat on the floor.
- Activate and tighten your abdominal muscles.
- Keep your eyes fixed straight ahead so that your neck and back are neutrally aligned.

Hints & Tips

- Activate your abdominals to maintain stability and a neutral posture with your shoulders back and chest out.
- Breathe out as you lift your arms. Breathe in as you lower them down.

forward hand walk

Areas Worked: Shoulders and core
Names of Main Muscle Groups: Anterior Deltoid, medial deltoid, posterior deltoid, and Transversus Abdominus

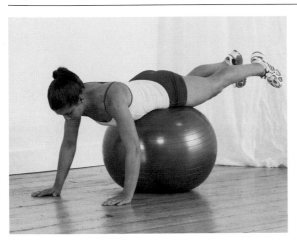

1 Lie face down on the Swiss Ball with your arms extended, hands on the floor and legs extended at the hip. Hold a neutral position with a straight line running from your shoulders to your ankles.

2 Walk your hands forward, rolling the ball underneath you until it reaches your feet.

3 Pause, and then walk your hands back, rolling the ball back underneath you until you reach the start position.

Technique

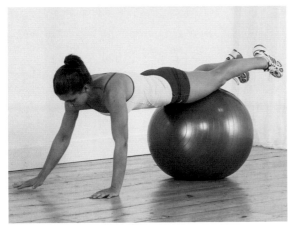

- Lie on the ball with your hips are resting on the center.
- Position your hands on the floor so that they are directly below your shoulders.
- Activate and tighten your core muscles to maintain a neutral position, with a straight line running from your shoulders to your ankles.
- Make sure that your back doesn't arch and your hips don't rotate during the exercise.
- Face the floor throughout the movement to keep your neck neutrally aligned.
- Lift, reach, and place your hands one at a time.
- Avoid locking your elbows when your arms are straight.

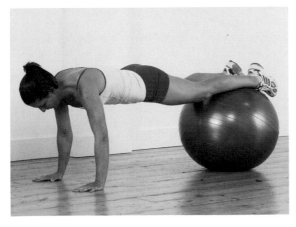

Hints & Tips

- The length your arm reaches will affect the difficulty of the exercise. Start with a short position reach and progressively increase the distance as you gain stability.
- Focus on keeping your body from neck to ankles in a straight line. Imagine that you are a ridged plank.

Balance and Stability
Advanced

kneeling shoulder press

Areas Worked: Front of shoulders, back of upper arms, and core
Names of Main Muscle Groups: Anterior Deltoid and Triceps

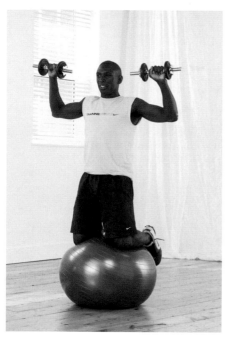 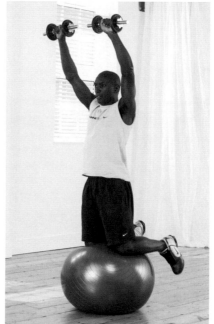

1 Take hold of a weight in both hands with an over-hand grip.

2 Kneel up on top of the ball.

3 Position the weights just above shoulder level.

4 Extend your arms, pushing the weights above your head.

5 Pause, and then flex your arms, lowering the weights back down to the start position.

Technique

- Place yourself directly in the center of the Swiss Ball.
- Your knees should be bent to 90 degrees.
- Activate and tighten your abdominal muscles as you straighten your back.
- Keep your eyes fixed straight ahead so that your neck and back are neutrally aligned.
- Start with your elbows pointed out to the side, keeping your forearms vertical.
- Lift your arms straight up so that they are vertical when fully extended.

Hints & Tips

- Practice getting on the ball in a kneeling position before doing the complete exercise.
- Activate your abdominals to adjust and maintain stability on the ball, and a neutral posture as you lift the weights above your head.
- Breathe out as you extend your arms. Breathe in as you lower them down.

kneeling lateral raise

Areas Worked: Top of shoulders and core
Names of Main Muscle Groups: Medial Deltoid, Upper Trapezius

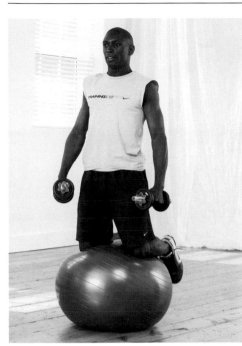

1 Take hold of a weight in both hands with an over-hand grip. Kneel up on top of the ball and position the weights down by your side.

2 Raise your arms up and out to the side until the weights are at shoulder height.

3 Pause, and then lower your arms returning the weights back down to the starting position.

Technique

- Place yourself directly in the center of the Swiss Ball.
- Your knees should be bent to 90 degrees.
- Activate and tighten your abdominal muscles as you straighten your back.
- Keep your eyes fixed straight ahead so that your neck and back are neutrally aligned.
- Ensure that your arms stay straight throughout the exercise.

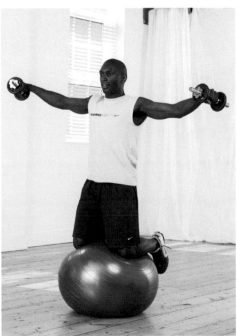

Hints & Tips

- Practice getting on the ball in a kneeling position before doing the complete exercise.
- Activate your abdominals to adjust and maintain stability on the ball, and a neutral posture as you lift your arms out to the side.
- Breathe out as you lift your arms. Breathe in as you lower them down.

kneeling front raise

Area Worked: Front of shoulders
Name of Main Muscle Group: Anterior Deltoid

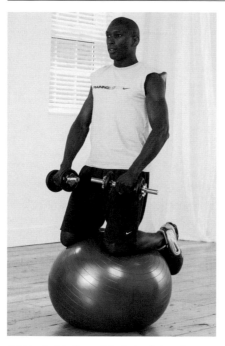 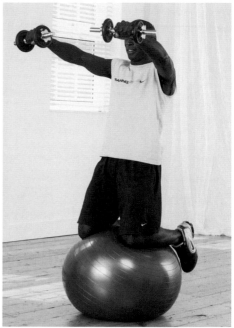

1 Take hold of a weight in both hands with an over-hand grip. Kneel on top of the ball. Position the weights down by your side.

2 Raise your arms forward and up until the weights are at shoulder height.

3 Pause, and then lower your arms, returning the weights back down to the start position.

Technique

- Place yourself directly in the center of the Swiss Ball.
- Your knees should be bent to 90 degrees.
- Activate and tighten your abdominal muscles as you straighten your back.
- Keep your eyes fixed straight ahead so that your neck and back are neutrally aligned.
- Ensure that your arms stay straight throughout the exercise.

Hints & Tips

- Practice getting on the ball in a kneeling position before doing the complete exercise.
- Activate your abdominals to adjust and maintain stability on the ball, and a neutral posture as you lift your arms forward.
- Breathe out as you lift your arms. Breathe in as you lower them down.

hand walk around

Areas Worked: Shoulders and core
Names of Main Muscle Groups: Anterior Deltoid, medial deltoid, posterior deltoid, and Transversus Abdominus

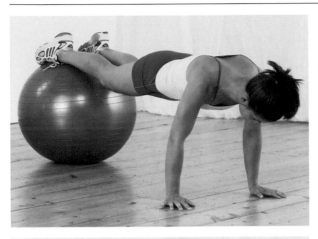

1 Position your hands on the floor so that they are directly below your shoulders. Your upper foot and shin should be resting against the top of the ball.
2 Lift, reach, and place your arms one at a time as you walk them around the ball.

Technique

- Place yourself directly in the center of the Swiss Ball.
- Your knees should be bent to 90 degrees.
- Activate and tighten your abdominal muscles as you straighten your back.
- Make sure that your back doesn't arch and your hips don't rotate during the exercise.
- Face the floor so that your neck and back are neutrally aligned.
- Ensure that your arms stay straight and avoid locking your elbows.

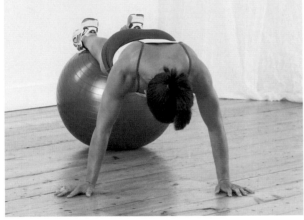

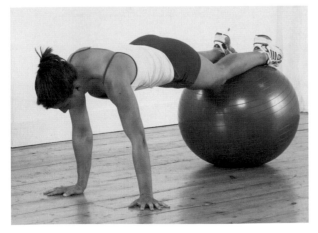

Hints & Tips

- The length your arm reaches will affect the difficulty of the exercise. Start with a short position reach and progressively increase the distance as you gain stability.
- Focus on keeping your body, from your neck to your ankles, in a straight line. Imagine that you are a ridged plank.

Arm Exercises
Strength and Tone
Beginner–Intermediate

seated bicep curls

Area Worked: Front of upper arm
Name of Main Muscle Group: Biceps

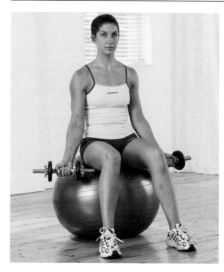 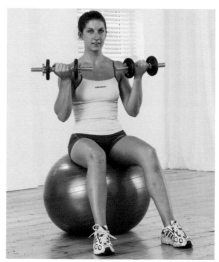

1 Sit on the ball with your feet flat on the floor. Take hold of a weight in both hands, with an under-hand grip, positioning them down by your side.

2 Flex your arms at the elbows, lifting the weights toward your shoulders.

3 Pause, and then extend your arms, lowering the weights back down to the start position.

Technique

- Position yourself on the center of the Swiss Ball.
- Bend your knees to 90 degrees.
- Activate and tighten your abdominal muscles, keeping your back straight.
- Keep your eyes fixed straight ahead so that your neck and back are neutrally aligned.
- Hold the weights straight as you flex and extend your arms.
- Ensure that your upper arms stay vertical and fixed by your sides.

Hints & Tips
- Keep your feet firmly planted on the floor to help you balance on the ball.
- Maintain the resistance against your biceps by stopping before the weight reaches your shoulders.
- Breathe out as you flex your arms. Breathe in as you extend them and lower the weight back down.

seated overhead triceps extension

Area Worked: Back of upper arm
Name of Main Muscle Group: Triceps

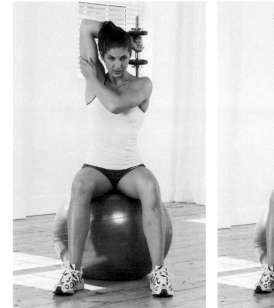 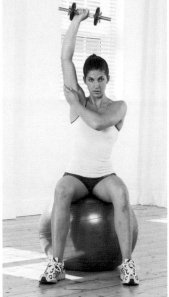

1 Sit on the ball with your feet flat on the floor. Take hold of a weight in one hand with an over-hand grip.

2 Extend your upper arm so that it is vertical and parallel to your head, with your elbow bent and weight dropped down toward the opposite shoulder.

3 Extend your arm, lifting the weight until your arm is straight.

4 Pause, and then flex your arm, lowering the weight back down toward your shoulder to the start position.

5 Repeat the exercise using your other arm.

Technique

- Place yourself directly in the center of the Swiss Ball.
- Your knees should be bent to 90 degrees.
- Activate and tighten your abdominal muscles.
- When in the start position the forearm of your active arm should be positioned behind your head.
- Keep your head as straight as possible so that you are not craning it forward.
- Extend your arm straight up so that it is vertical, when fully extended, but not fully locked.

Hints & Tips

- Start with your inactive arm around the front of the opposite shoulder to support the active arm, and prevent your upper arm from moving as you flex and extend it.
- Keep your feet firmly planted on the floor for balance.
- Activate your abdominals to maintain stability and a neutral posture as you extend your arm above your head.
- Breathe out as you extend your arm. Breathe in as you lower it down.

wrist extension

Areas Worked: Back of wrist and forearm
Name of Main Muscle Group: Wrist Extensors

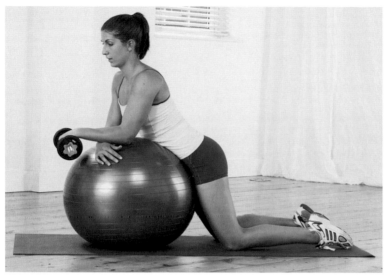

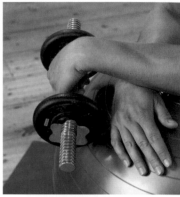

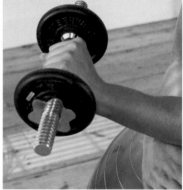

1 Kneel down on the floor, leaning against the Swiss Ball.

2 Take hold of a weight with your left hand using an over-hand grip; keeping your arm flexed, rest your elbow on top of the ball.

3 Place your right arm across the top of the ball with your hand resting under your left forearm.

4 Extend your left wrist, pulling your hand back toward you.

5 Pause, and then lower your hand back down to the start position.

6 Repeat the exercise using your right hand and reversing the placement of your arms.

Technique

- Position yourself with your hips pressed into the ball.
- Activate and tighten your abdominal muscles, holding your back straight and your shoulders high.
- Position the weight lowered toward the ball before starting the exercise.
- Hold the weight straight as you extend your wrist.
- Ensure that your forearm stays fixed in position throughout the movement.

Hints & Tips

- Press your elbow into the ball to keep your arm still and to isolate your wrist.
- Control the level of your shoulders with the static arm keeping them straight.
- Breathe out as you extend your wrist. Breathe in as you flex it and lower the weight back down.

wrist flexion

Areas Worked: Front of wrist and forearm
Name of Main Muscle Group: Wrist Flexors

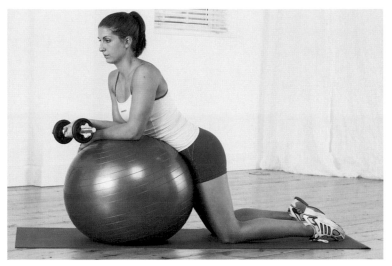

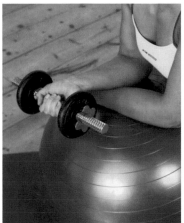

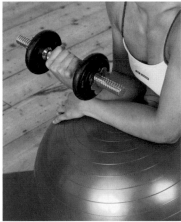

1 Kneel down on the floor, leaning against the Swiss Ball.

2 Take hold of a weight with your right hand, using an under-hand grip. Keep your arm flexed and rest your elbow on top of the ball.

3 Place your left arm across the top of the ball with your hand resting under your right forearm.

4 Flex your right wrist, pulling your hand up toward you.

5 Pause, and then lower your hand back down to the start position.

6 Repeat the exercise using your left side and reversing the placement of your arms.

Technique

- Position yourself with your hips pressed into the ball.
- Activate and tighten your abdominal muscles, holding your back straight and shoulders high.
- Position the weight lowered toward the ball before you start the exercise.
- Hold the weight straight as you flex your wrist.
- Ensure that your forearm arm stays fixed in position throughout the movement.

Hints & Tips

- Press your elbow into the ball to keep your arm still and to isolate your wrist.
- Control the level of your shoulders with the static arm keeping them straight.
- Breathe out as you flex your wrist. Breathe in as you extend it and lower the weight back down.

Strength and Tone
Advanced

bicep preacher curls

Area Worked: Front of upper arm
Name of Main Muscle Group: Biceps

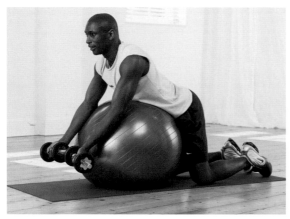 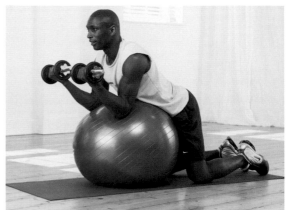

1 Kneel down on the floor, leaning against the Swiss Ball.

2 Take hold of a weight in both hands with an underhand grip, arms extended and elbows resting against the ball.

3 Flex your arms at the elbows, lifting the weights toward your shoulders.

4 Pause, and then extend your arms, lowering the weights back down to the start position.

Technique

- Position yourself with your hips pressed into the ball.
- Activate and tighten your abdominal muscles, holding your back straight and your shoulders high.
- Start with your arms straight and palms facing upward.
- Hold the weights straight as you flex your arms.
- Ensure that your upper arms stay fixed in position throughout the movement.

Hints & Tips

- Press your elbows into the ball to keep your upper arm still and to isolate your biceps.
- Breathe out as you flex your arms. Breathe in as you extend them and lower the weights back down.

single arm bicep preacher curl

Area Worked: Front of upper arm
Name of Main Muscle Group: Biceps

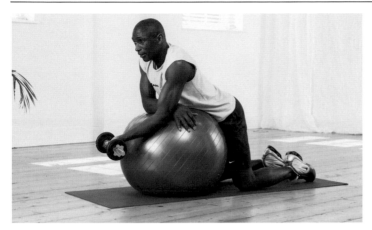

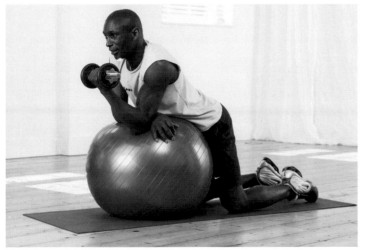

1 Kneel down on the floor, leaning against the Swiss Ball. Take hold of a weight with your left hand, using an under-hand grip. Extend your arm with your elbow resting against the ball.

2 Place your right arm across the top of the ball with your hand behind your left elbow.

3 Flex your left arm at the elbow, lifting the weight toward your left shoulder.

4 Pause, and then extend your arm, lowering the weight back down to the start position.

5 Repeat the exercise using your right arm.

Technique

- Position yourself with your hips pressed into the ball.
- Activate and tighten your abdominal muscles, holding your back straight and your shoulders high.
- Start with your active arm straight and palm facing upward.
- Hold the weight straight as you flex your arm.
- Ensure that your upper arm stays fixed in position throughout the movement.

Hints & Tips

- Press your elbow into the ball to keep your upper arm still and to isolate your biceps.
- Control the level of your shoulders with the static arm keeping them straight.
- Maintain the resistance against your biceps by stopping the movement when the weights reach shoulder height.
- Activate your abdominals to maintain stability and a neutral posture, with your shoulders back and chest out.
- Breathe out as you flex your arm. Breathe in as you extend it and lower the weight back down.

75

tricep dips

Area Worked: Back of upper arms
Name of Main Muscle Group: Triceps

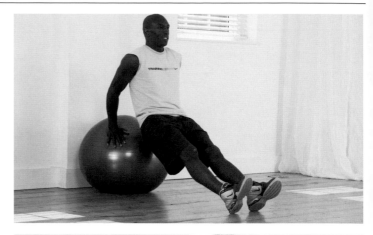

1 Place the Swiss Ball against the wall. With the ball behind you, position your hands on top of it with your arms straight, and stretch out your legs in front of you so that your heels are on the floor.

2 Bend your arms, dropping your bottom toward the floor, until your elbows are at a 90-degree angle.

3 Pause, and then extend your arms, lifting yourself away from the floor and back to the start position.

Technique

- Keep your hips flexed and your legs extended throughout the movement.
- Activate and tighten your core muscles, to hold your back neutrally and in a vertical position, as you flex and extend your arms.
- Pivot on your heel as you lower and raise yourself on the ball.
- Your elbows should stay parallel to each other as you bend your arms, keeping your forearms vertical.
- Stop at the bottom of the movement, when you feel a stretch across the front of your shoulders.

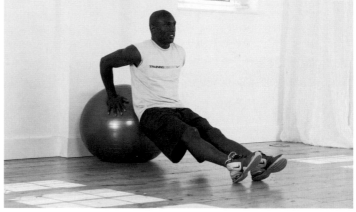

Hints & Tips

- Position your hands on the front edge of the ball to give yourself room to move up and down in front of it.
- Increase the flexion in your hips as you lower yourself down to assist with keeping your back straight.
- You can make it easier by bending your knees slightly and placing your feet flat on the floor.
- Breathe in as you bend your arms and lower yourself down, breathe out as you extend your arms and push yourself back up.

Balance and Stability
Beginner–Intermediate–Advanced

seated bicep curls, leg extended

Areas Worked: Front of upper arm and core
Name of Main Muscle Group: Biceps

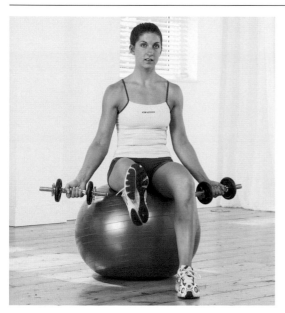

1. Sit on the ball with your feet flat on the floor. Take hold of a weight in both hands with an under-hand grip, positioning them down by your side. Extend one leg off the floor.

2. Flex your arms at the elbows, lifting the weights toward your shoulders.

3. Pause, and then extend your arms, lowering the weights back down to the start position.

4. Repeat, using your other leg.

Technique

- Position yourself on the center of the Swiss Ball.
- Bend one knee to 90 degrees with your foot on the floor.
- Hold your extended leg off the floor for the duration of the exercise.
- Activate and tighten your abdominal muscles, holding your back straight.
- Keep your eyes fixed straight ahead so that your neck and back are neutrally aligned.
- Hold the weights straight as you flex and extend your arms.

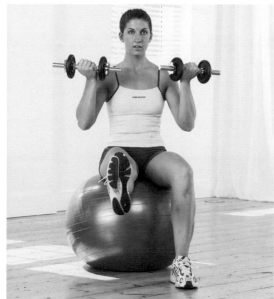

Hints & Tips

- Fix your upper arms by your sides, stopping them from moving back and forth as you flex your arms.
- Keep one foot firmly planted on the floor to help you balance on the ball.
- Maintain the resistance against your biceps by stopping the movement before the weight reaches your shoulders.
- Activate your abdominals to maintain stability and a neutral posture, with your shoulders back and chest out.
- Breathe out as you flex your arms. Breathe in as you extend them and lower the weight back down.

seated overhead triceps, leg extended

Areas Worked: Back of upper arm and core
Name of Main Muscle Group: Triceps

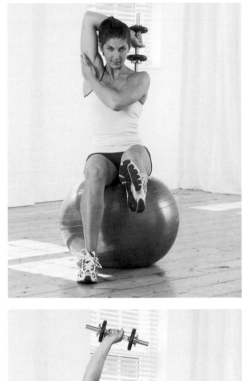

1 Sit on the ball with one foot flat on the floor. Take hold of a weight in one hand with an over-hand grip.

2 Extend your upper arm so that it is vertical and parallel to your head, with your elbow bent and weight dropped down toward the opposite shoulder.

3 Lift and extend one leg off the floor.

4 Extend your arm, lifting the weight until your arm is straight.

5 Pause, and then flex your arm, lowering the weight back down toward your shoulder and the start position.

6 Repeat the exercise with your other arm, and other leg extended.

Technique

- Place yourself directly in the center of the Swiss Ball.
- The knee of your stabilizing leg should be bent to 90 degrees.
- Your other leg should remain extended straight for the duration of the exercise.
- When in the start position the forearm of your active arm should be positioned behind your head.
- Keep your head as straight as possible so that you are not craning it forward.
- Extend your arm straight up so that it is vertical when fully extended.

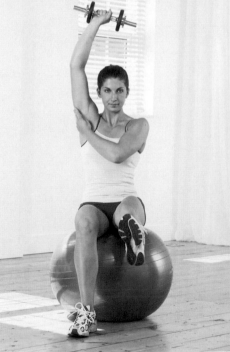

Hints & Tips

- Start with your inactive arm around the front of the opposite shoulder to support the active arm, and prevent your upper arm from moving as you flex and extend it.
- Keep the foot of your stabilizing leg firmly planted on the floor for balance.
- Activate your abdominals to maintain stability and a neutral posture as you extend your arm above your head.
- Breathe out as you extend your arm. Breathe in as you lower it down.

triceps french press

Areas worked: Back of upper arm and core
Name of Main Muscle Group: Triceps

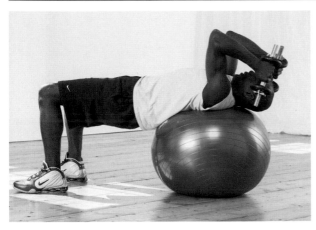

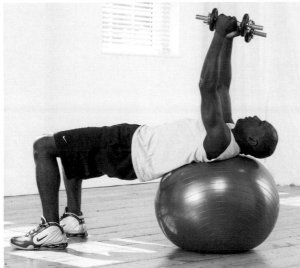

1 Lie on your back on top of the ball in the reverse bridge position, with your knees bent at 90 degrees. Take hold of a dumbbell in each hand, with a palms-in grip.

2 Position your upper arms so that they are vertical, with your elbows flexed and weights toward the level of your shoulders.

3 Extend both arms, pushing the weights up, until they are straight.

4 Pause and then slowly bend your arms, allowing them to return back toward your shoulders.

Technique

- The ball should be positioned so that it sits directly between your shoulder blades.
- Place your feet shoulder width apart.
- Activate and tighten your abdominal muscles to help maintain a neutral alignment.
- Be careful not to let your pelvis drop and move out of alignment. You should form a straight line from your shoulders through to knees.
- Stop at the bottom of the movement when you feel a stretch in your triceps.

Hints & Tips

- As you hold your upper arms vertically, make sure that they stay parallel with each other.
- Ensure that the weights are positioned wide enough apart as you flex your elbows in order to avoid hitting yourself on the head as they are lowered down.
- Your foot position has a huge impact on how difficult the exercise is with regards to stability. The closer your feet are together the less stable you will be. Start by placing them shoulder width apart; as you improve, gradually bring them closer together.
- Breathe out as you extend your arms. Breathe in as you return.

Lower Body Exercises
Strength and Tone
Beginner–Intermediate

squat against wall

Areas Worked: Front of upper legs and bottom
Names of Main Muscle Groups: Quadriceps and Gluteus Maximus

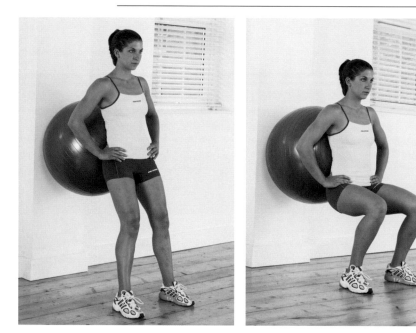

1 Place the Swiss Ball against the wall and lean your lower back into it.

2 Stand with feet shoulder width apart.

3 Flex your hips and your knees, lowering your buttocks down toward the floor and rolling the ball up your back.

4 Pause and then extend your hips and knees. Lift yourself straight and back to the start position.

Technique

- Start with your legs straight, feet placed ahead of the ball and parallel to each other, and back neutrally aligned as you rest against the ball.
- Activate and tighten your abdominal muscles, tilting pelvis forward slightly to help maintain a neutral alignment as you flex your hips and knees.
- Look straight ahead and keep your shoulders back as you lower yourself down.
- Stop at the bottom of the movement just before your knees reach a 90-degree angle.
- Keep your back in contact with the ball throughout the exercise.

Hints & Tips

- Start with the ball positioned against your lower back and upper pelvis so that it rides up your back and supports it correctly throughout the movement.
- Keep your heels in contact with the floor throughout the exercise. Push through them to assist your hips and knees as you extend them.
- Breathe in as you flex your knees and lower yourself down. Breathe out as you extend your knees.

squat and ball hold

Areas Worked: Front of upper legs, buttocks, and core
Names of Main Muscle Groups: Quadriceps and Gluteus Maximus

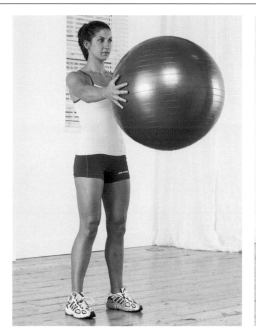 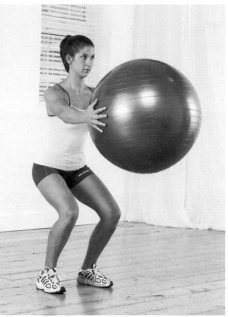

1 Stand with feet shoulder width apart.
2 Take hold of the Swiss Ball with your hands on either side of it and extend arms in front of you.
3 Flex your hips and your knees, lowering yourself back and down.
4 Pause and then extend your hips and knees, lifting yourself straight and back to the start position.

Technique

- Start with your legs straight, feet parallel, and back neutrally aligned.
- Position your arms so that they are straight and parallel to the floor, holding them there for the duration.
- Activate and tighten your abdominal muscles, tilting the pelvis forward slightly to help maintain a neutral alignment as you flex your hips and knees.
- Look straight ahead and keep your shoulders back as you lower yourself down.
- Stop at the bottom of the movement, just before your knees reach a 90-degree angle.

Hints & Tips

- Shift your body weight back onto your heels as you lower yourself down, using an action as if you were about to sit down on a chair.
- Keep your heels in contact with the floor throughout the exercise, push through them to assist your hips and knees as you extend them.
- Breathe in as you flex your knees and lower yourself down. Breathe out as you extend your knees.

seated leg extension

Areas Worked: Front of upper leg and core
Name of Main Muscle Group: Quadriceps

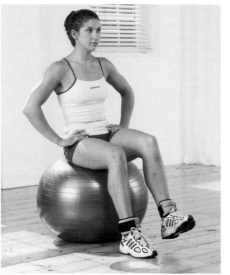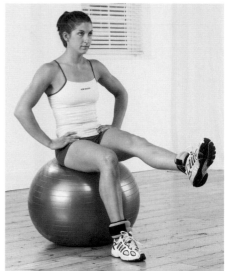

1 Place an ankle weight around each ankle.

2 Sit on the ball with your right foot flat on the floor, and left foot raised off the floor slightly.

3 Extend your left knee, lifting your foot until your leg is straight.

4 Pause, and then flex your left knee, lowering your foot back down to the starting position.

5 Repeat using your other leg.

Technique

- Position yourself on the center of the Swiss Ball.
- Bend one knee to 90 degrees with your foot on the floor.
- Activate and tighten abdominal muscles, holding your back straight and stabilizing yourself on the ball.
- Keep your eyes fixed straight ahead so that your neck and back are neutrally aligned.
- Extend your knee and lift your foot until your leg is straight and horizontal.

Hints & Tips

- Place your hands on your hips to help keep your shoulders level.
- Keep one foot firmly planted on the floor to help you balance on the ball.
- Maintain the resistance against your quadriceps by stopping your foot before it touches the floor.
- Activate your abdominals to maintain stability and a neutral posture, with your shoulders back and chest out.
- Breathe out as you extend your knee. Breathe in as you flex your knee.

prone hamstring curls

Area Worked: Back of upper legs
Name of Main Muscle Group: Hamstrings

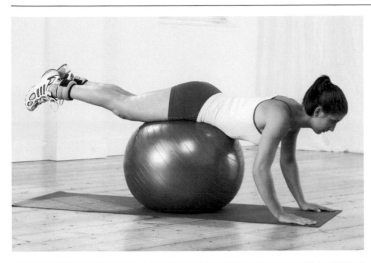

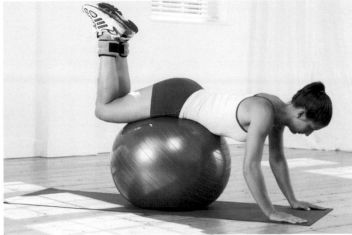

1 Secure an ankle weight around each ankle.

2 Lie prone on the Swiss Ball with arms extended, hands on the floor, and legs extended straight.

3 Flex your knees, lifting your feet up.

4 Pause, and then extend your legs, lowering your feet back down to the start position.

Technique

- Lie on the ball with your hips resting on the center.
- Position your hands on the floor so that they are directly below your shoulders.
- Hold a neutral position with a straight line running from your shoulders to your knees.
- Make sure that your back doesn't arch and your hips don't flex during the exercise.
- Keep your knees and feet together as you flex your knees.
- Flex your knees from straight legs to a 90-degree angle.

Hints & Tips

- Stop the flexion when the lower part of your legs are vertical.
- Use slow controlled movements to get the most from the exercise.
- Breathe out as you flex your knees. Breathe in as you extend your knees.

side to side jumping

Areas Worked: Front of upper leg, back of lower leg, buttocks, and outer thigh
Name of Main Muscle Groups: Quadriceps, Gastrocnemius/Soleus, Gluteus Maximus, and Gluteus Medius

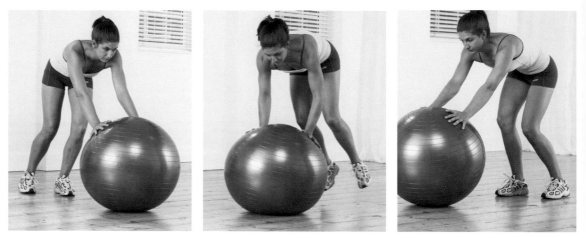

Technique

- Position feet hip width apart.
- Flex at the hips and lean forward, placing your hands on top of the ball.
- Pivot the ball with your hands as you jump from one side to the other.
- Keep your arms extended throughout the exercise.

1 Stand behind and to the side of the Swiss Ball, with feet flat on the floor and hands on top of the ball.

2 Stabilizing your upper body with your arms, jump your feet across to the other side of the ball.

3 As soon as your feet touch the floor, jump back to the starting position.

4 Continue this movement for the desired number of repetitions.

Hints & Tips

- Position your hands wide apart on the ball to assist stability.
- Fix your eyes on the spot where you are wanting to jump to. This will help you to keep the jump distances consistent as you have a point to aim for.
- Progressively increase the distance of your jumps as you gain stability, strength, and power.

side lying outer thigh

Area Worked: Outer thigh (Hip abductor)
Name of Main Muscle Group: Gluteus Medius

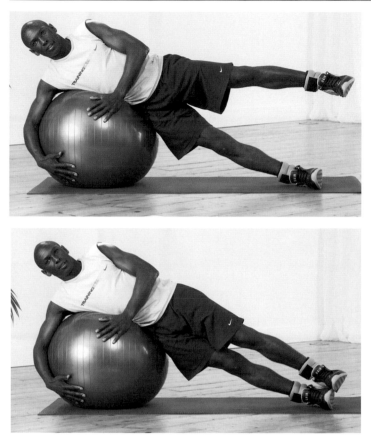

1 Lie on your right-hand side against the Swiss Ball, legs extended, with the outside of your right foot on the floor.

2 Abduct your left hip, lifting your leg up and out to the side.

3 Pause, and slowly lower your left leg, dropping your foot toward the other and returning back to the starting position.

Technique

- Keep your upper body still, with your shoulders and hips vertically aligned as you abduct your hip.
- Both legs should be straight throughout the movement.
- Aim to get the active leg horizontal at the top of the movement.

Hints & Tips

- Keep the resistance against the hip abductors for the duration of the exercise by not touching your feet together at the bottom of the movement.
- Balance your weight position on the ball with the leg that is in contact with the floor.
- Breathe out as you lift your leg. Breathe in as you lower your leg back down.

inner thigh ball press

Area Worked: Inner thigh
Name of Main Muscle Group: Adductors

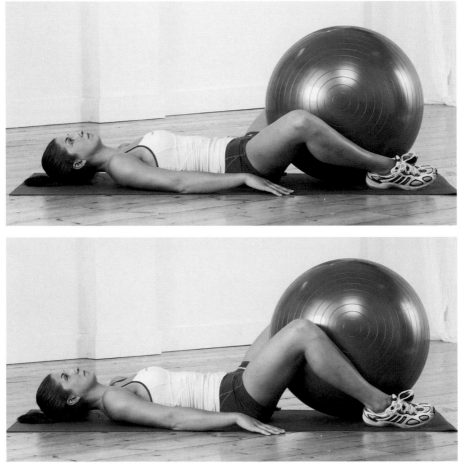

1 Position yourself lying on your back on the floor, with knees bent.

2 Place the ball between your legs.

3 Adduct your hips, and squeeze the ball between your knees.

4 Hold for 4 seconds, and then relax your hips.

Technique

- Activate and tighten your core muscles to maintain a neutral back position on the floor.
- Position the ball between your legs, flexed to a 90-degree angle, so that the ball is in contact with your knees and lower legs.
- Make sure that your back doesn't arch and that your feet remain on the floor during the exercise.

Hints & Tips

- Squeeze your knees together putting equal pressure on the ball as if trying to burst it.
- Allow the ball to push your legs back out as you relax, keeping them in contact with it at all times.
- Breathe out as you adduct your hips. Breathe in as you relax.

Strength and Tone
Advanced

squat on ball

Areas Worked: Front of upper legs, buttocks, and core
Names of Main Muscle Groups: Quadriceps and Gluteus Maximus

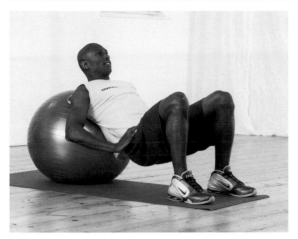 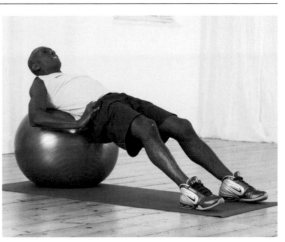

1 Lie with your back against the Swiss Ball and your knees bent at 90 degrees, feet shoulder width apart. Drop your hips down until your torso is at a 45-degree angle.

2 Extend your hips and knees, rolling yourself up on the ball.

3 Pause, and then flex your hips and knees, lowering your buttocks down toward the floor and back to the start position.

Technique

- Activate and tighten your abdominal muscles to help maintain a neutral alignment as you extend your hips and knees.
- Form a straight line from your ankles to your shoulders when your legs and hips are fully extended.
- Look straight ahead and keep your shoulders back as you lower yourself down.
- Stop at the bottom of the movement, just before your knees reach a 90-degree angle.

Hints & Tips

- Start with the ball positioned between your shoulder blades, so that it rolls down your back and supports it correctly throughout the movement.
- Keep your heels in contact with the floor throughout the exercise, push through them to assist your hips and knees as you extend them.
- The closer your feet are together, the less stable you will be.
- Breathe out as you extend your knees. Breathe in as you lower yourself down.

single leg squat against wall

Areas Worked: Front of upper legs, buttocks, and core
Names of Main Muscle Groups: Quadriceps and Gluteus Maximus

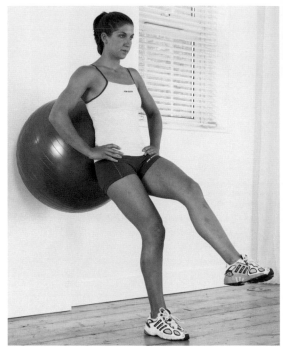

1 Place the Swiss Ball against the wall and lean your lower back into it.

2 Stand on your right leg, with your leg extended.

3 Flex your right hip and knee, lowering your buttocks down toward the floor and rolling the ball up your back.

4 Pause, and then extend your right hip and knee, pushing yourself straight and back to the start position.

Technique

• Lean your back against the ball with your right leg straight and foot placed ahead of the ball.

• Extend your left leg and hold your foot off the floor.

• Activate and tighten your abdominal muscles, tilting your pelvis forward slightly to help maintain a neutral alignment, as you flex your hip and knee.

• Look straight ahead and keep your shoulders back as you lower yourself down.

• Stop at the bottom of the movement, just before your knee reaches a 90-degree angle.

• Keep your back in contact with the ball throughout the exercise.

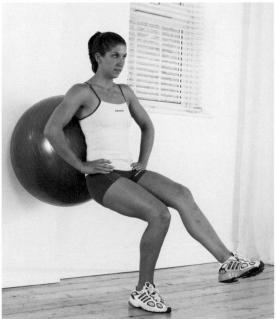

Hints & Tips

• Start with the ball positioned against your lower back and upper pelvis so that it rides up your back and supports it correctly throughout the movement.

• Keep the heel of your active leg in contact with the floor throughout the exercise, and push through it to assist your hip and knee as you extend them.

• Use your core muscles to balance as you change your position on the ball.

• Breathe in as you flex your knees and lower yourself down. Breathe out as you extend your knees.

hamstring curls

Areas Worked: Back of upper legs and core
Name of Main Muscle Group: Hamstrings

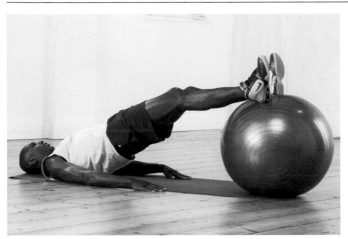

1 Position yourself lying on your back on the floor, with heels resting on top of the ball.

2 Extend your hips so that you are in the reverse bridge position and hold.

3 Flex your knees, pulling your heels toward your buttocks.

4 Pause, and then extend your knees, dropping them down and straightening your legs back to the start position.

Technique

- Start in the bridge position, forming a straight line from your shoulders to your ankles. Only the back of your shoulders should be in contact with the floor.
- Activate and tighten your core muscles to maintain the neutral position.
- Make sure that your back doesn't arch during the exercise.
- Flex your knees until they are at a 90-degree angle. In this position you should be maintaining a straight line from your shoulders to your knees.

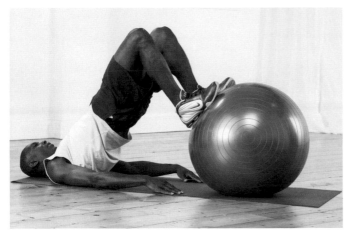

Hints & Tips

- Place your hands on the floor by your sides to assist with stability.
- Roll the ball from your heels to the balls of your foot for a smooth movement.
- Breathe out as you flex your knees. Breathe in as you extend your knees.

side lying inner thigh

Area Worked: Inner thigh
Name of Main Muscle Group: Adductors

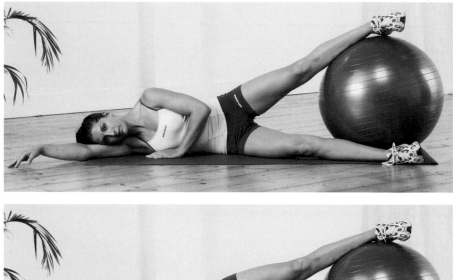

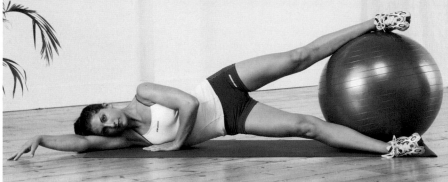

1 Lie on the floor on your right-hand side. Lift your left leg and rest it on top of the Swiss Ball.

2 Adduct your left hip against the ball, lifting your pelvis off the floor.

3 Pause, and then slowly lower your pelvis back down, returning to the starting position.

4 Repeat the exercise on your other side.

Technique

- Keep your upper body stable with your shoulders and hips vertically aligned as you adduct your hip.
- Rest the weight of your upper body onto the shoulders as your pelvis lifts, keeping your back straight throughout the movement.
- Aim to get the active leg horizontal at the top of the movement.

Hints & Tips

- Place your inactive leg on the floor in front of the ball to help keep your balance.
- Keep the resistance against the hip abductors for the duration of the exercise by not resting your pelvis down completely between repetitions.
- Breathe out as you adduct your hip. Breathe in as you relax back down.

Balance and Stability
Beginner–Intermediate

reverse bridge single leg extension

Areas Worked: Front of upper leg and core
Name of Main Muscle Group: Quadriceps

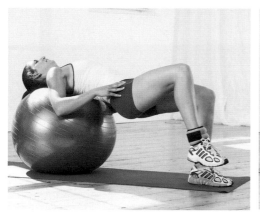

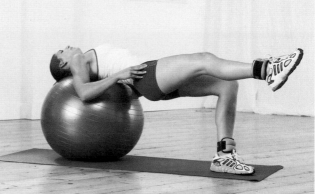

1 Attach an ankle weight around each ankle.

2 Lie on your back on top of the ball in the reverse bridge position, with your knees bent at 90 degrees and your right foot elevated off the floor slightly.

3 Extend your right knee, lifting your foot until your leg is straight.

4 Pause, and then flex your knee, lowering your foot back down toward the floor.

5 Repeat the exercise using your left leg.

Technique

- The ball should be positioned so that it sits directly between your shoulder blades.
- Activate and tighten your abdominal muscles to help maintain a neutral alignment.
- Stabilize your weight with the foot that is on the floor.
- Keep your upper leg static and horizontal as you extend and flex your knee.
- Stop at the bottom of the movement when your knee reaches a 90-degree angle.

Hints & Tips
- Place your hands on your hips during the exercise to keep your upper body position balanced.
- Focus on creating a straight line from your hip to your ankle when you extend your knee.
- Breathe out as you extend your knee. Breathe in as you flex your knee.

reverse bridge single hip flexion

Areas worked: Front of hip and core
Name of Main Muscle Group: Psoas

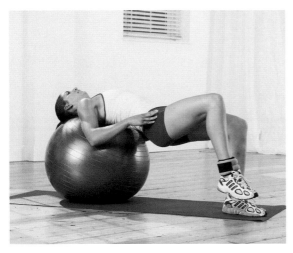
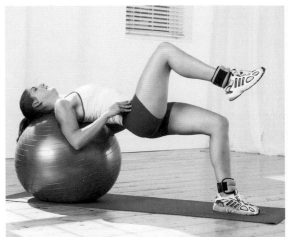

1 Attach an ankle weight around each ankle.

2 Lie on your back on top of the ball in the reverse bridge position, with your knees bent at 90 degrees and your right foot elevated off the floor slightly.

3 Flex your right hip, lifting your knee and foot up.

4 Pause, and then extend your hip, lowering your knee and foot back down toward the floor.

5 Repeat the exercise using your left leg.

Technique

- The ball should be positioned so that it sits directly between your shoulder blades.
- Activate and tighten your abdominal muscles to help maintain a neutral alignment.
- Stabilize your weight with the foot that is on the floor.
- Keep the knee bent at 90 degrees for the duration of the exercise to isolate your hip.
- Stop at the bottom of the movement, just before your foot touches the floor.

Hints & Tips

- Place your hands on your hips during the exercise to keep your upper body position balanced.
- When flexing your hip, stop at the top of the movement, just before your upper leg reaches a vertical position. This keeps tension against the hip flexor muscles.
- Breathe out as you flex your hip. Breathe in as you extend your hip.

bridge

Areas Worked: Buttocks, back of upper legs, and core
Names of Main Muscle Groups: Gluteus Maximus and Hamstrings

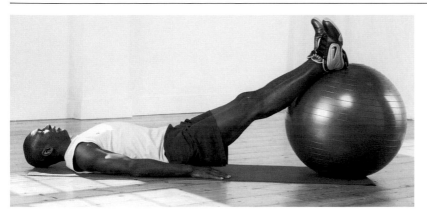

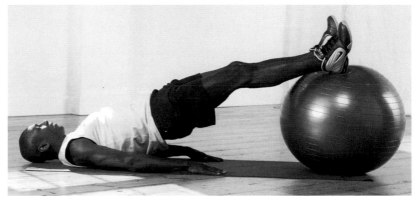

1 Position yourself lying on your back on the floor, with heels resting on top of the ball.

2 Extend your hips, lifting your buttocks off the floor.

3 Hold at the top of the movement for 3 seconds, and then flex your hips, dropping your buttocks back down toward the floor.

Technique

- Start with your feet on the ball, your buttocks just off the floor, so you aren't resting your full weight down.
- Lift your pelvis up by extending your hips so that only the back of your shoulders are in contact with the floor.
- Activate and tighten your core muscles to maintain the neutral position with a straight line from your shoulders to your hips.
- Make sure that your back doesn't arch during the exercise.

Hints & Tips

- Place your hands on the floor by your sides to assist with stability.
- Breathe out as you extend your hips. Breathe in as you flex your hips and lower your buttocks down.

prone single hip extensions

Areas Worked: Buttocks and back of upper leg
Names of Main Muscle Groups: Gluteus Maximus and Hamstrings

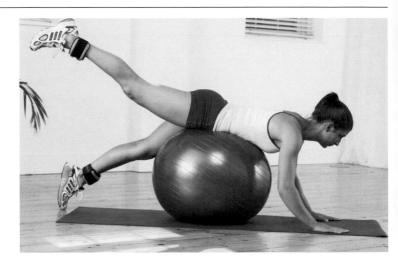

1 Secure an ankle weight around each ankle.

2 Lie prone on the Swiss Ball with arms slightly bent, hands on the floor, and your right leg extended just above the floor.

3 Extend your right hip, lifting your leg up.

4 Pause, and then flex your right hip, lowering your leg back down to the starting position.

5 Repeat, using your left hip.

Technique

- Lie on the ball with your hips resting on the center of the top of the ball.
- Position your hands on the floor so that they are just ahead of your shoulders.
- Lift the toes of the leg and hip, which you are about to extend, a few inches off the floor.
- Rest the toes of your inactive leg on the floor for stability.
- Hold a neutral position in your back and hold it in position throughout the exercise.
- Keep both legs straight as you extend one hip at a time.

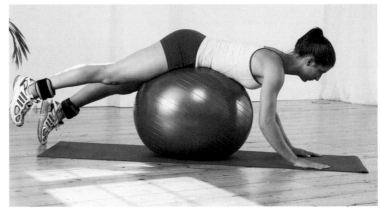

Hints & Tips

- Extend your hip and lift your leg as high as you can without arching your back.
- Stop the flexion of your hip just before toes touch the floor.
- Use slow controlled movements to get the most from the exercise.
- Breathe out as you extend your hip. Breathe in as you flex your hip and lower your leg.

prone bent knee and hip extensions

Areas Worked: Buttocks and back of upper leg
Names of Main Muscle Groups: Gluteus Maximus and Hamstrings

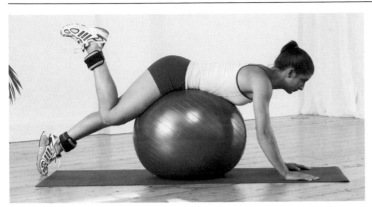

1 Secure an ankle weight around each ankle.

2 Position yourself prone on the Swiss Ball with arms extended, hands on the floor, and your right leg flexed to 90 degrees.

3 Extend your right hip, lifting your leg up.

4 Pause, and then flex your right hip, lowering your leg back down to the starting position.

5 Repeat, using your left hip.

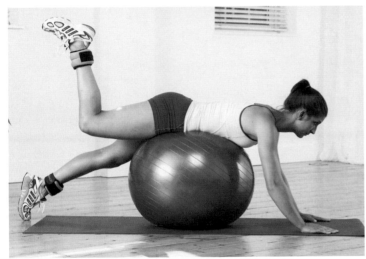

Technique

- Lie on the ball with your hips resting on the center of the top of the ball.
- Position your hands on the floor so that they are just ahead of your shoulders.
- Flex the knee of the leg that you are about to work to a 90-degree angle and hold it in that position with your thigh resting gently against the ball.
- Hold a neutral position in your back and hold it in position throughout the exercise.

Hints & Tips

- Rest the toes of your inactive leg on the floor for stability.
- Extend your hip and lift your leg as high as you can, imagining that you are trying to push your heel up into the ceiling.
- Flex your hip back down but not resting all of its weight onto the ball.
- Use slow controlled movements to get the most from the exercise.
- Breathe out as you extend your hip. Breathe in as you flex your hip back down.

reverse bridge leg rotations

Areas Worked: Front of hip, inner and outer thigh
Names of Main Muscle Groups: Psoas, Gluteus Medius, and Adductors

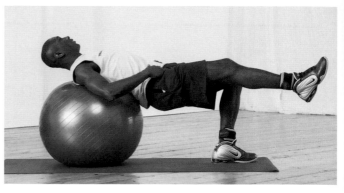

1 Attach an ankle weight around each ankle.

2 Lie on your back on top of the ball in the reverse bridge position, with your left knee bent at 90 degrees and your right foot elevated off the floor with your leg straight.

3 Rotate your leg at the hip, creating circles with your foot in a clockwise direction.

4 Pause, and then circle your foot in a counterclockwise direction.

5 Repeat the exercise using your left leg.

Technique

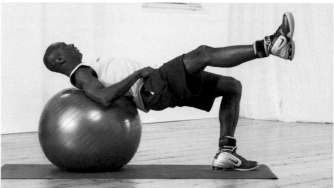

- The ball should be positioned so that it sits directly between your shoulder blades.
- Activate and tighten your abdominal muscles to help maintain a neutral alignment.
- Stabilize your weight with the foot that is on the floor.
- Hold your active leg straight as you make circles with your foot.

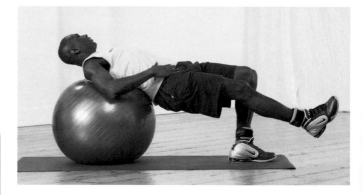

Hints & Tips

- Place your hands on your hips during the exercise to keep your upper body position balanced.
- Focus on creating a straight line from your hip to your ankle when you extend your knee.
- Progressively increase the size of the circle that you make with your foot to make the exercise more difficult.

Balance and Stability
Advanced

single leg squat on ball

Areas Worked: Front of upper legs, buttocks, and core
Names of Main Muscle Groups: Quadriceps and Gluteus Maximus

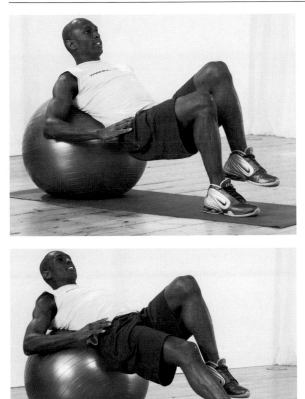

1 Lie your back against the Swiss Ball, with your right knee bent to 90 degrees and foot on the floor.

2 Drop your hips down until your torso is at a 45-degree angle.

3 Bend your left leg and flex your hip, holding your foot off the floor.

4 Extend your left hip and knee, rolling yourself up on the ball.

5 Pause, and then flex your hip and knee, lowering your buttocks down toward the floor and back to the start position.

6 Repeat using your left leg with your right foot off the floor.

Technique

- Activate and tighten your abdominal muscles to help maintain your balance as you extend your hip and knee.
- Form a straight line from your ankle to your shoulder when your leg and hip are fully extended.
- Look straight ahead and keep your shoulders back as you lower yourself down.
- Stop at the bottom of the movement just before your knee reaches a 90-degree angle.

Hints & Tips

- Start with the ball positioned between your shoulder blades, so that it rolls down your back and supports it correctly throughout the movement.
- Keep the heel of your active leg in contact with the floor throughout the exercise. Push through it to assist your hip and knee as you extend them.
- Breathe out as you extend your knees. Breathe in as you lower yourself down.

standing single leg squat

Areas Worked: Front of upper leg, buttocks, and core
Names of Main Muscle Groups: Quadriceps and Gluteus Maximus

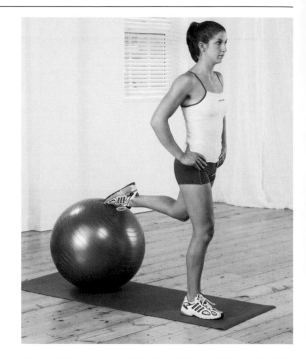

1 Stand with the Swiss Ball on the floor behind you.

2 Balance your weight on your right leg. Lift your left foot and place it on top of the ball behind you.

3 Flex your right hip and knee, lowering your buttocks down toward the floor.

4 Pause, and then extend your right hip and knee, pushing yourself straight and back to the start position.

5 Repeat, standing on your left leg, with your right foot on the ball.

Technique

- Position the ball a couple of feet behind you.
- Rest the toe of the elevated leg on the center of the top of the ball.
- Activate and tighten your abdominal muscles, tilting pelvis forward slightly to help maintain a neutral alignment as you flex your hip and knee.
- Look straight ahead and keep your shoulders back as you lower yourself down.
- Stop at the bottom of the movement, just before your knee reaches a 90-degree angle.
- Keep shoulders high as you flex your knee and hip.

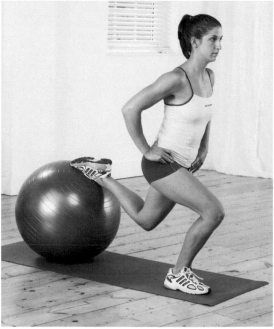

Hints & Tips

- Take time to control your balance before starting the exercise.
- Keep the heel of your active leg in contact with the floor throughout the exercise. Push through it to assist your hip and knee as you extend them.
- Use your core muscles to balance as your back leg looks for stability on the ball.
- Breathe in as you flex your knees and lower yourself down. Breathe out as you extend your knees.

single leg hamstring curls

Areas Worked: Back of upper leg and core
Name of Main Muscle Group: Hamstrings

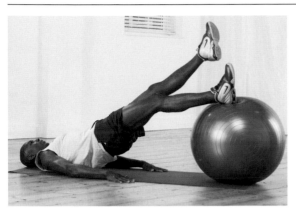

1 Position yourself lying on your back on the floor, with your right heel resting on top of the ball, and your left leg elevated.

2 Extend your hips so that you are in the reverse bridge position and hold.

3 Flex your right knee, pulling your heel toward your buttocks.

4 Pause, and then extend your right knee, dropping it down and straightening your leg back to the start position.

5 Repeat the exercise with your left heel on the ball and your right leg elevated.

Technique

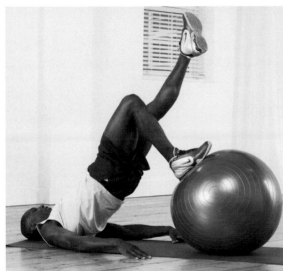

- Start in the bridge position, forming a straight line from your shoulders to your ankle. Only the back of your shoulders should be in contact with the floor.
- Activate and tighten your core muscles to maintain the neutral position.
- Make sure that your back doesn't arch during the exercise.
- Hold the inactive leg straight and above the ball so that it doesn't make contact with it.
- Flex the knee of your active leg until it is at a 90-degree angle. In this position you should be maintaining a straight line from your shoulders to your knee.

Hints & Tips

- Place your hands on the floor by your sides to assist with stability.
- Roll the ball from your heel to the ball of your foot for a smooth movement.
- Breathe out as you flex your knee. Breathe in as you extend your knee.

single leg bridge

Areas Worked: Buttocks, back of upper legs, and core
Names of Main Muscle Groups: Gluteus Maximus and hamstrings

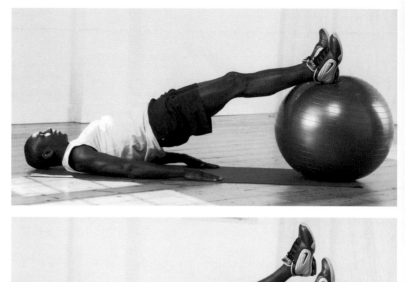

1 Position yourself lying on your back on the floor, with heels resting on top of the ball.

2 Extend your left hip, lifting your buttocks off the floor. At the same time, flex your right hip, lifting your heel away from the ball.

3 Hold at the top of the movement for 3 seconds and then flex your left hip, dropping your buttocks back down toward the floor.

4 Repeat the exercise, extending your right hip against the ball.

Technique

- Start with your feet on the ball, your buttocks just off the floor, so that you are not resting your full weight down.

- Lift your pelvis up by extending one hip, whilst lifting your other heel off the ball by flexing the hip of the same leg, with all the resistance being controlled by the heel that is on the ball.

- Only the back of your shoulders should be in contact with the floor at the top of the movement.

- Activate and tighten your core muscles to maintain the neutral position with a straight line from your shoulders to your hip.

- Make sure that your back doesn't arch during the exercise.

Hints & Tips

- Place your hands on the floor by your sides to assist with stability.
- Breathe out as you extend your hips. Breathe in as you flex your hips and lower your buttocks down.

prone hip extensions

Areas worked: Buttocks and back of upper legs
Names of Main Muscle Groups: Gluteus Maximus and hamstrings

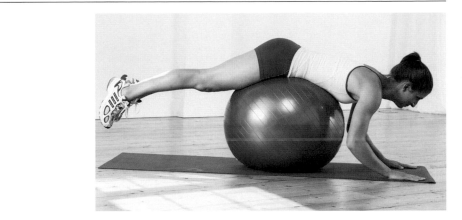

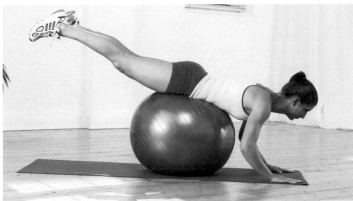

1 Secure an ankle weight around each ankle.

2 Lie prone on the Swiss Ball with arms slightly bent, hands on the floor, and leg extended just above the floor.

3 Extend your hips, lifting both legs up together.

4 Pause, and then flex your hips, lowering your legs back down to the starting position.

Technique

- Lie on the ball with your hips resting on the center of the top of the ball.
- Position your hands on the floor so that they are just ahead of your shoulders.
- Hold a neutral position in your back and hold it in position throughout the exercise.
- Keep your legs straight, with knees and feet together, as you extend your hips.

Hints & Tips

- Extend your hips and lift your legs as high as you can without arching your back.
- Stop the flexion of your hips just before your toes touch the floor.
- Use slow controlled movements to get the most from the exercise.
- Breathe out as you extend your hips. Breathe in as you flex your hips and lower your legs.

Midsection Exercises
Strength and Tone
Beginner–Intermediate

abdominal crunch basic

Area Worked: Abdomen
Name of Main Muscle Group: Rectus Abdominus

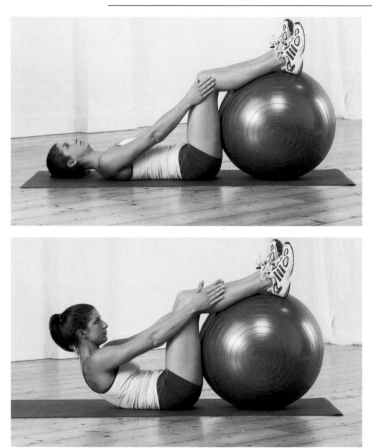

1 Lie on your back on the floor, with your legs flexed and your heels resting on top of the ball.

2 Roll your shoulders forward, lifting them off the floor.

3 Hold at the top of the movement for 3 seconds, and then relax back down toward the floor.

Technique

- Start with your legs flexed to 90-degrees and your feet on the ball.
- Position your hands on the outside of each knee when you extend your arms.
- Activate and tighten your abdominal muscles to roll and lift your shoulders forward as you reach your hands toward your ankles.
- Make sure that only your shoulders lift away from the floor, and not your back.

Hints & Tips

- Placing your hands on the sides of your legs and reaching them toward your ankles gives you a consistent point to aim for. Also ensure that you lift your shoulders and flex your abdomen through the correct range of movement.
- Breathe out as you roll your shoulders forward. Breathe in as you relax back down.

abdominal curl on ball

Area Worked: Abdomen
Name of Main Muscle Group: Rectus Abdominus

1 Lie on the Swiss Ball with your knees bent at 90 degrees.

2 Extend your arms with your hands on top of your thighs.

3 Raise your shoulders away from the ball.

4 Hold for 3 seconds and then slowly lower your shoulders back to the start position.

Technique

- Position yourself so that your mid back and upper pelvis are resting against the ball.
- Place your feet shoulder width apart.
- Drop your pelvis down slightly so that it is pressing into the ball as you raise your shoulders.
- Activate and tighten your abdominal muscles to flex your midsection and lift your shoulders forward as you reach your hands toward your knees.
- Stop at the bottom of the movement just before your shoulders touch down on the ball.

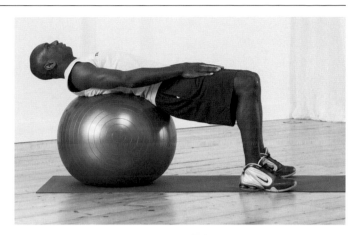

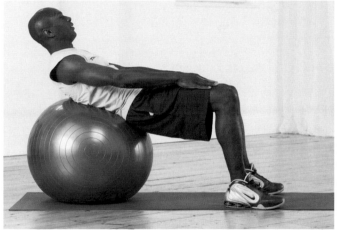

Hints & Tips

- Sliding your hands on top of your legs toward your knees will give you a consistent point to aim for as you lift your shoulders.
- Keep constant resistance against your abdominals by not resting your weight down completely between repetitions.
- Breathe out as you roll your shoulders forward. Breathe in as you relax back down.

abdominal curl rotation

Areas Worked: Abdomen and sides of midsection
Names of Main Muscle Groups: Rectus Abdominus and External Obliques

1 Lie on the Swiss Ball, with your knees bent at 90 degrees.

2 Extend your right arm, with your hand on top of your left thigh.

3 Reach your right arm along your thigh and raise and rotate your upper body and shoulders toward the left and away from the ball.

4 Hold for 3 seconds and then slowly lower yourself down, straightening your shoulders back to the start position.

5 Repeat, using your left arm and rotating toward the right.

Technique

• Position yourself so that your mid back and upper pelvis are resting against the ball.

• Place your feet shoulder width apart.

• Drop your pelvis down slightly so that it is pressing into the ball as you raise your shoulders.

• Activate and tighten your abdominal muscles, to flex and rotate your midsection and lift your shoulder forward, as you reach your hand toward your knee.

• Stop at the bottom of the movement, just before your shoulders touch down on the ball.

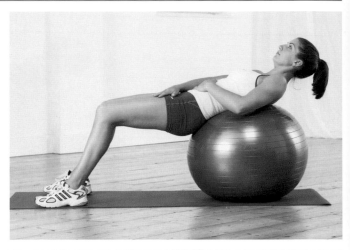

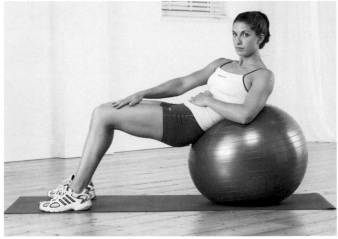

Hints & Tips

• Slide your hand on top of your opposite leg, toward your knee, in a constant and smooth movement.

• Keep constant resistance against your abdominals by not resting your weight down completely between repetitions.

• Breathe out as you raise your shoulders and rotate your torso. Breathe in as you relax back down.

reverse curl

Area Worked: Lower abdomen
Name of Main Muscle Group: Rectus Abdominus

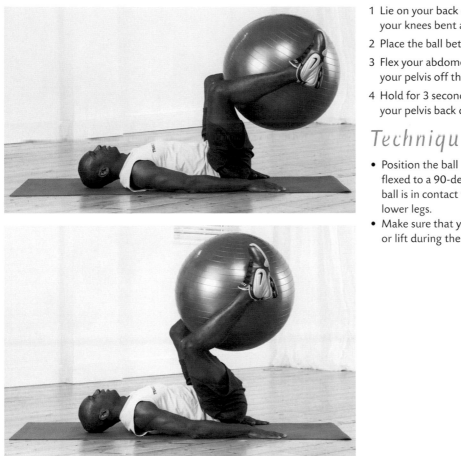

1 Lie on your back on the floor, with your knees bent and your feet raised.

2 Place the ball between your legs.

3 Flex your abdomen, tilting and lifting your pelvis off the floor.

4 Hold for 3 seconds, and then lower your pelvis back down.

Technique

- Position the ball between your legs, flexed to a 90-degree angle, so that the ball is in contact with your knees and lower legs.
- Make sure that your back doesn't arch or lift during the exercise.

Hints & Tips

- Hollow your abdominals and pull your pelvis back, tilting it off the floor.
- Keep your back and shoulders firmly placed on the floor to isolate the lower region.
- Your legs should remain fixed in position so that they follow the movement of your pelvis.
- Breathe out as you tilt and lift your pelvis. Breathe in as you relax.

back extension/torso rotation with toes on floor

Areas Worked: Lower back and sides of midsection
Names of Main Muscle Groups: Erector Spinae and External Obliques

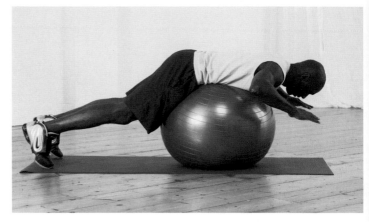

1 Lie face down on the Swiss Ball, so that your navel is on the center of the ball, and your legs are extended.

2 Extend your back, lifting your chest away from the ball, and rotate your torso to the right.

3 Pause, and then lower your chest and shoulders back down to the ball and the start position.

4 Repeat, extending your back and rotating your torso to the left.

Technique

• Keep your legs extended straight behind you, with your toes on the floor.

• Hold your arms out at a 90-degree angle to your body with your elbows bent.

• As you extend your back slowly rotate your torso, so that you are looking out to the side.

• Hold your hips square on to the ball as you rotate.

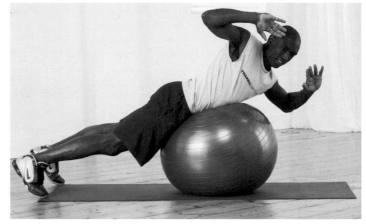

Hints & Tips

• Squeeze your shoulder blades together and pull your arms back as you extend and rotate.

• Push your hips into the ball as you lift your chest away.

• To help you to rotate your torso imagine that you are aiming to point one elbow to the floor and the other to the ceiling while keeping them parallel to each other.

• Breathe out as you extend your back and rotate. Breathe in as you lower your chest back down to the ball.

Strength and Tone
Advanced

weighted abdominal curl

Area Worked: Abdomen
Name of Main Muscle Group: Rectus Abdominus

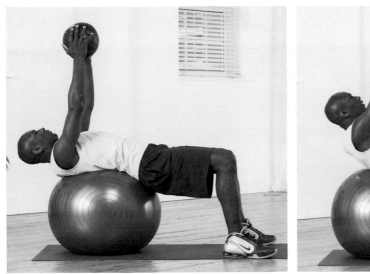 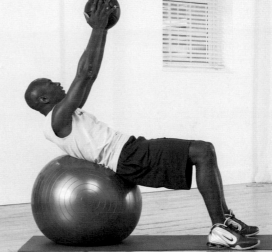

1 Lie on the Swiss Ball, with your knees bent at 90 degrees.

2 Take hold of the medicine ball and extend your arms up.

3 Raise your shoulders away from the Swiss Ball.

4 Hold for 3 seconds and then slowly lower your shoulders back to the start position.

Technique

- Position yourself so that your mid back and upper pelvis are resting against the ball.
- Place your feet shoulder width apart.
- Drop your pelvis down slightly so that it is pressing into the ball as you raise your shoulders.
- Activate and tighten your abdominal muscles to flex your midsection and lift your shoulders forward, keeping your arms and the medicine ball up.
- Stop at the bottom of the movement, just before your shoulders touch down on the ball.

Hints & Tips

- Start with your arms straight and vertical with your hands either side of the medicine ball. Fix them in position, so that as you lift your shoulders the ball moves up and forward adding additional resistance to the exercise.
- Keep constant resistance against your abdominals by not resting your weight down completely between repetitions.
- Breathe out as you roll your shoulders forward. Breathe in as you relax back down.

lying curl and flex

Areas Worked: Abdomen and sides of midsection
Names of Main Muscle Groups: Rectus Abdominus and External Obliques

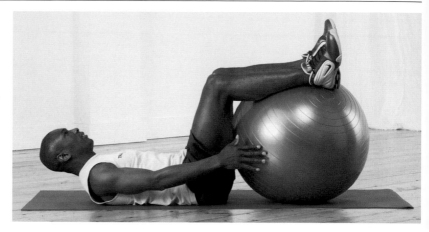

1 Lie with your back on the floor, your knees bent and your heels resting on top of the Swiss Ball.

2 Flex your abdomen, lifting your shoulders from the floor slightly.

3 Flex your midsection, reaching your right hand to the side of the ball.

4 Pause, and then flex the other way, positioning your body straight again.

5 Repeat, flexing your midsection to the left.

Technique

• Lie with your back flat on the floor.

• Position your lower legs with them flexed to a 90-degree angle, and so that your lower leg and heels are resting on top of the ball.

• Start with your finger tips resting on the sides of the ball, and then aim to reach them as far around the outside edge as possible.

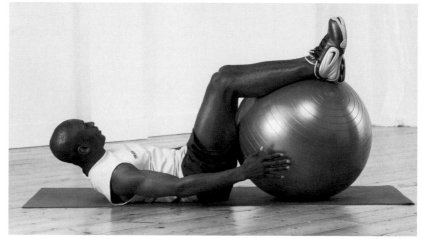

Hints & Tips

• To get the most from the exercise, keep your abdominals flexed slightly, with your shoulders raised off the floor for the duration of the exercise.

• Keep your legs fixed in position throughout the movement.

• Breathe out as you reach around the ball. Breathe in as you relax.

ball raise lateral flexion

Area Worked: Sides of midsection
Name of Main Muscle Groups: External Obliques and Quadratus Lumborum

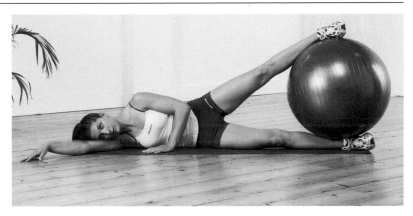

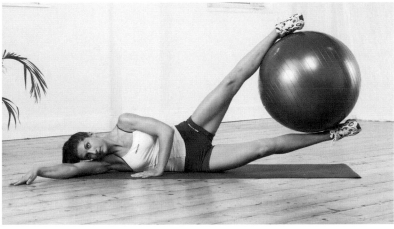

1 Lie on the floor on your right-hand side, gripping the Swiss Ball between your ankles.

2 Flex your midsection, lifting your legs and ball away from the floor.

3 Pause, and then slowly lower your pelvis back down, returning to the start position.

4 Repeat the exercise on your other side.

Technique

- Keep your upper body stable, with your shoulders and hips vertically aligned as you adduct your hip.
- Rest the weight of your upper body onto your shoulder and side as you flex your midsection.
- Aim to lift your legs as high as you can at the top of the movement.

Hints & Tips

- Use the arm of the shoulder that is away from the floor to support your position by placing the hand on the floor in front of you.
- Keep a strict form by using slow controlled movements.
- Breathe out as you laterally flex your midsection. Breathe in as you relax back down.

Balance and Stability
Beginner–Intermediate

sitting on the ball

Area Worked: Core
Name of Main Muscle Group: Transversus Abdominus

1 Sit on the ball with your feet flat on the floor.

2 Extend your arms and legs forward.

3 Hold and balance for 10 second intervals.

Technique

- Place yourself directly in the center of the Swiss Ball.
- Activate and tighten your abdominal muscles.
- Keep your eyes fixed straight ahead so that your neck and back are neutrally aligned.
- Extend your arms and legs straight so that they are not in contact with the floor.

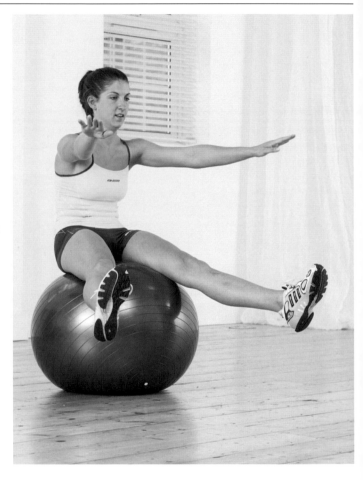

Hints & Tips

- Correct your position on the ball to gain stability.
- Activate your abdominals to maintain stability and a neutral posture while your arms and legs are extended.

lying lateral flexion

Area Worked: Sides of midsection
Names of Main Muscle Groups: External Obliques and Quadratus Lumborum

1 Lie on your left-hand side against the Swiss Ball, legs extended and feet on the floor.

2 Flex your midsection, lifting your pelvis away from the floor.

3 Pause, and slowly lower your pelvis, returning back to the start position.

Technique

- Position yourself against the ball so that it is in contact with the side of your rib cage.
- Your legs should be straight, with your feet staggered.
- Bend both arms, resting one over the ball and the other on the side.
- Start with your midsection flexed toward the floor.
- Lift your pelvis away from the floor as you flex, until your body and legs form a straight line.
- Activate and tighten your abdominal muscles to help maintain a neutral back position.

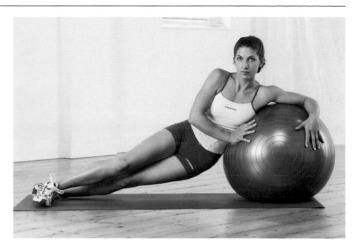

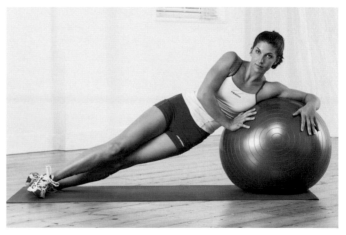

Hints & Tips

- Stabilize your shoulders and hip in a vertical position so that you can focus on the lateral flexion of your midsection.
- As you are laterally flexing your midsection, push your side into the ball, working the muscles harder.
- Stagger the placement of your feet, one in front of the other, to keep yourself balanced.
- Breathe out as you lift your pelvis away from the floor. Breathe in as you lower yourself back down.

reverse bridge ball rolls

Areas Worked: Midsection, sides of midsection, and core
Names of Main Muscle Groups: Transversus Abdominus, Internal Obliques, and External Obliques

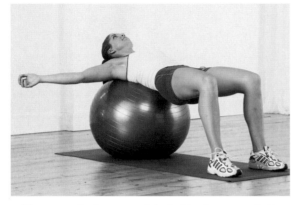
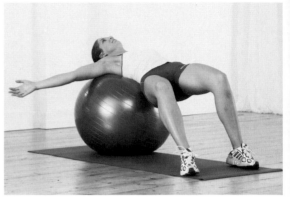

1 Lie on your back on top of the ball in the reverse bridge position, with your knees bent at 90 degrees.

2 Position your arms out to the side.

3 Move your upper body across the ball to the right, rolling the ball under your shoulders and toward your right shoulder.

4 Pause, and then slowly roll the ball back to the center of your shoulders.

5 Repeat the exercise, rolling your shoulders across the ball the other way, under your left shoulder.

Technique

• Start with the ball positioned so that it sits directly between your shoulder blades.

• Place your feet shoulder width apart.

• Activate and tighten your abdominal muscles to help maintain a neutral alignment.

• Be careful not to let your pelvis drop and move out of alignment. You should form a straight line from your shoulders through to your knees.

• Hold your arms out to the side, so that they are straight, and your hands level with your shoulders.

• Laterally flex your midsection, moving your shoulders across the top of the ball as it about to roll off completely, keeping your feet flat on the floor.

Hints & Tips

• Hold your body stable as you roll across the ball, working against the rotation that the ball is trying to induce.

• Stop moving off the ball when it is lying directly under one shoulder.

• Progressively increase the size of your upper body flexion on the ball as you become more stable.

• Your foot position has a large impact on how difficult the exercise is with regards to stability. The closer your feet are together the less stable you will be. Start by placing them shoulder width apart. As you improve, gradually bring them closer together.

• Breathe out as you roll on the ball. Breathe in as you return.

reverse bridge torso rotation

Areas Worked: Sides of midsection and core
Names of Main Muscle Groups: Internal and External Obliques

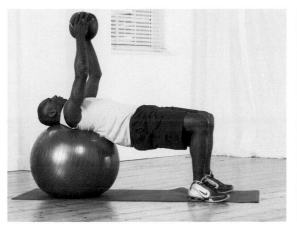 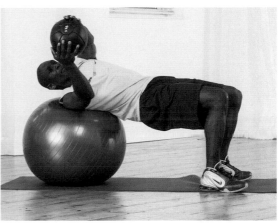

1 Lie on your back on top of the ball in the reverse bridge position, with your knees bent at 90 degrees.

2 Take hold of the medicine ball with both hands, and position your arms straight up.

3 Rotate your upper body to the right, rolling onto your shoulder on top of the ball.

4 Pause, and then slowly roll back with the Swiss Ball in the center of your shoulders.

5 Repeat the exercise, rotating your torso and rolling on your shoulder the other way.

Technique

- Start with the ball positioned so that it sits directly between your shoulder blades.
- Place your feet shoulder width apart.
- Activate and tighten your abdominal muscles to help maintain a neutral alignment.
- Form a straight line from your shoulders through to your knees.
- Hold onto the medicine ball with your arms up, so that they are vertical, and level with your shoulders.
- Keep your arms straight throughout the movement, arcing the ball over as you roll onto your shoulder.

Hints & Tips

- Keep your hips in line with your knees as you rotate your upper body, to work your spinal rotators.
- Hold your body stable as you rotate your torso on the ball, working against the instability induced by the ball.
- Stop rotating when the ball is lying directly under one shoulder and your shoulders are vertical.
- Progressively increase the size of your torso rotations on the ball as you become more stable and gain mobility.
- Your foot position has a large impact on how difficult the exercise is with regards to stability. The closer your feet are together the less stable you will be. Start by placing them shoulder width apart, bringing them closer together as you improve.
- Breathe out as you rotate on the ball. Breathe in as you return.

Balance and Stability
Advanced

transverse abs

Area Worked: Core
Name of Main Muscle Group: Transversus Abdominus

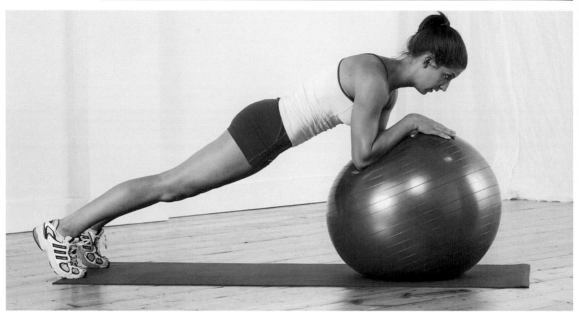

1 Position yourself on your toes with your arms bent and forearms resting on top of the ball.

2 Hold a straight line from your ankles to your shoulders.

3 Maintain this position for as long as you can.

Technique

- Position your shoulders over your elbows so that they are vertical.
- Activate and tighten your core muscles to maintain a neutral position, with a straight line running from your shoulders to your ankles.

Hints & Tips

- Hold the position, stopping before your pelvis drops out of line and your back arches.
- Your foot position will also affect the difficulty of the exercise. Closer to the ball is harder.
- Control a normal breathing pattern throughout the exercise.

transverse abs, leg elevated

Area Worked: Core
Names of Main Muscle Groups: Transversus Abdominus and Internal Obliques

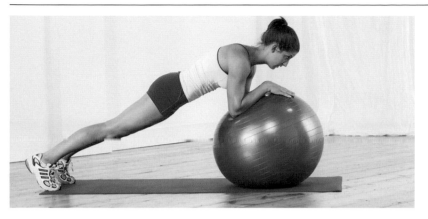

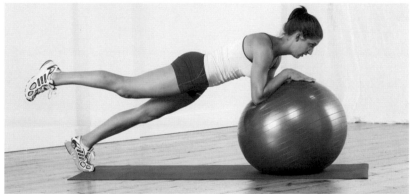

1 Position yourself on your toes with your arm bent and your forearms resting on top of the ball.

2 Maintain a straight line from your ankles to your shoulders then lift your right leg away from the floor.

3 Hold for 5 seconds and then repeat, lifting your left leg away from the floor.

4 Continue the alternate leg lifts and holds for the desired number of repetitions.

Technique

- Position your shoulders over your elbows so that they are vertical.
- Activate and tighten your core muscles to maintain a neutral position, with a straight line running from your shoulders to your ankles.
- Prevent your pelvis from tilting or rotating as you lift your leg away from the floor.

Hints & Tips

- Hold the position, stopping before your pelvis drops out of line and your back arches.
- Your foot position will also affect the difficulty of the exercise. In this case wider apart is harder.
- Breathe normally throughout the exercise.

jack knife

Areas Worked: Lower abdomen and front of hips, with upper body and core stabilization
Names of Main Muscle Groups: Rectus Abdominus, Rectus Femoris, Psoas, and Transversus Abdominus

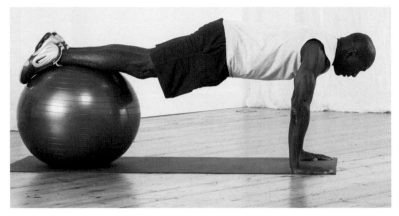

1 Support yourself on your hands, with your arms and legs extended and your toes resting on top of the Swiss Ball.

2 Hold a neutral position, with a straight line running from your shoulders to your ankles.

3 Flex your hips and bend your knees, pulling them in toward your body.

4 Pause, and extend your hips, taking your legs straight again, and back to the start position.

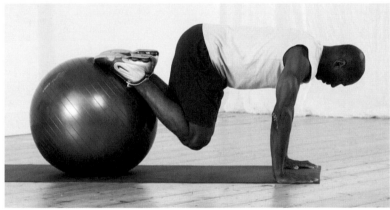

Technique

- Position your hands on the floor so that they are directly below your shoulders.
- The top of your foot and shin should be resting against the top of the ball.
- Make sure that your back doesn't arch as you flex your hips.
- Flex your hips and bend your knees until your thighs are vertical.
- Face the floor throughout the movement to keep your neck neutrally aligned.

Hints & Tips

- Activate and tighten your core muscles to hold a straight line from your shoulders to your ankles, and control your midsection as you flex your hips.
- Breathe out as you flex your hips. Breathe in as you extend your hips.

kneeling on the ball

Area Worked: Core
Name of Main Muscle Group: Transversus Abdominus

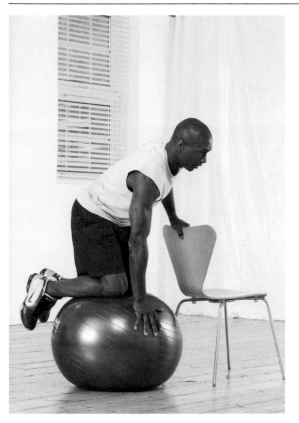 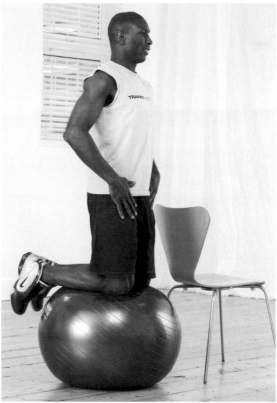

1 Stand behind the Swiss ball and place your hands and then knees on top of the ball.

2 Slowly lift your hands away and shoulders up until your torso is vertical.

3 Hold the position for as long as you are able to.

Technique

- Take your time in placing your hands and knees on the ball.
- Use a chair next to you to hold onto initially as you lift your hands away and your knees up.
- Activate and tighten your abdominal muscles to help maintain a neutral back position.

Hints & Tips

- Position yourself away from any hazardous objects, providing space in case you fall off the ball.
- Constantly adjust your position on the ball to gain stability.
- Most of all, be patient as this one takes time to master.

117

kneeling wood chop

Area Worked: Core
Name of Main Muscle Group: Transversus Abdominus

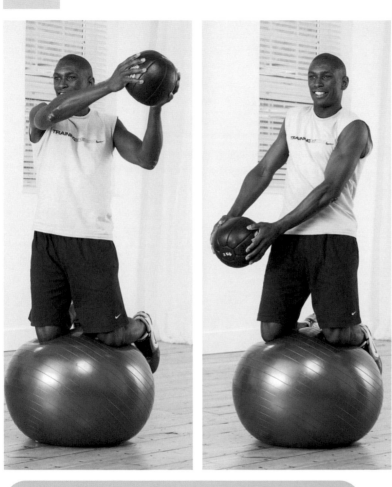

1 Kneel on the Swiss Ball, holding onto a medicine ball.
2 Start with the ball raised up and above your left shoulder.
3 Bring the ball down and across your body to the outside of your right hip.
4 Repeat, starting from your right shoulder, to your left hip.

Technique

- Position yourself in the center of the Swiss Ball.
- Activate and tighten your abdominal muscles, holding your back straight and stabilizing yourself on the ball.
- Keep your eyes fixed straight ahead so that your neck and back are neutrally aligned.
- Start by holding the ball above your shoulder with the arm that is across your body angled at 45 degrees to the opposite shoulder.
- Lower the ball down following the 45-degree angle and extending your arms until the medicine ball reaches the outside of your opposite hip.

Hints & Tips

- You should be competent at kneeling on the ball before attempting this exercise.
- The action resembles chopping a tree with an axe, so follow that same movement but with total control.
- Continuously adjust your balance as you displace your weight with the chopping action.
- Breathe out as you lower the medicine ball across your body. Breathe in as you raise the ball above your shoulder.

20-Minute Exercise Routines

Make sure that you have warmed up and stretched correctly, using the exercises in the Warm Up/Cool Down section, before starting any of the 20-minute Swiss Ball exercise routines listed below.

Having warmed up, start the first exercise, completing the first set of designated repetitions (progressively increasing the exercise intensity and range of movement). Rest for 30 seconds and then complete your second set. When all of your sets for each exercise are complete, rest for 40–60 seconds, and then move on to the next exercise. Continue in this way until you have completed all the exercises in this workout. It is advisable to perform a cool down and stretch after the workout is complete.

Always check with your doctor before starting any exercise routine.

Total Body Stability Routine – Beginner

press ups, kneeling on the floor

Sets: 2
Repetitions: 12–15
Areas Worked: Chest, front of shoulders, back of upper arms, and core

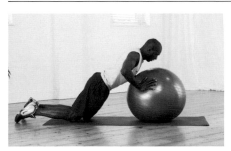

1 Kneel on the floor, leaning forward with your arms extended and your hands resting on top of the ball.

2 Bend your arms, bringing your chest toward the ball until your elbows reach 90 degrees.

3 Pause, and then extend your arms, pushing your chest away from the ball and returning to the start position.

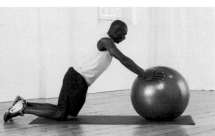

Technique

- Activate and tighten your abdominal muscles to help maintain a neutral back position.
- Pivot on your knees as you lower your upper body toward the ball.
- Your elbows should move out to the side as you bend your arms.
- Stop at the bottom of the movement, when you feel a stretch across your chest and shoulders.

mid row, leg extended

Sets: 2
Repetitions: 12–15
Areas Worked: Upper back, between the shoulder blades, back of shoulders, front of upper arms, and core

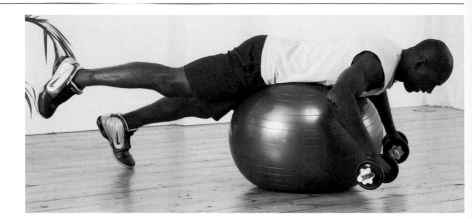

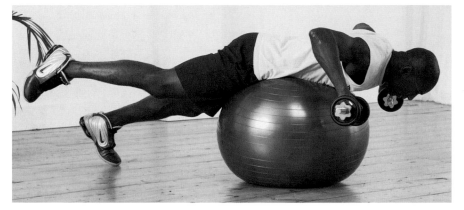

1 Lie face down on the Swiss Ball, with your right leg elevated off the floor, and the toes of your left leg on the floor.

2 Start with your upper arms out to the side and extended down toward the floor, holding the weights with an over-hand grip.

3 Lift your elbows up past shoulder level, bending your arms.

4 Pause, and then extend your arms, returning the weights back toward the floor.

5 Repeat, elevating your left leg.

Technique

- Hold your leg extended and foot off the floor for the duration of the exercise.
- Focus on control and keeping balanced as you lift the weights.
- Position your elbows out to the side at a 90-degree angle as you flex your arms.
- Stop at the bottom of the movement, making sure that the weights don't touch the floor.
- Ensure that your forearms are vertically positioned throughout the exercise.
- Keep your torso still during the movement.
- Make sure that your shoulders do not lift away from the ball as you raise your elbows.

forward hand walk

Sets: 2
Repetitions: 8–10
Areas Worked: Shoulders and core

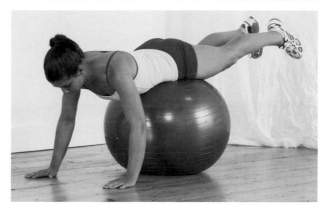

1 Lie face down on the Swiss Ball with your arms extended, hands on the floor, and legs extended at the hip.

2 Walk your hands forward, rolling the ball underneath you until it reaches your feet.

3 Pause and walk your hands back, rolling the ball back underneath you until you reach the start position.

Technique

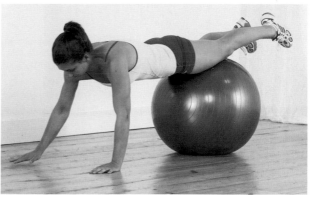

- Lie on the ball with your hips resting on the center.
- Position your hands on the floor so that they are directly below your shoulders.
- Activate and tighten your core muscles to maintain a neutral position with a straight line running from your shoulders to your ankles.
- Make sure that your back doesn't arch and your hips don't rotate during the exercise.
- Face the floor throughout the movement to keep your neck neutrally aligned.
- Lift, reach, and place your hands one at a time.
- Avoid locking your elbows when your arms are straight.

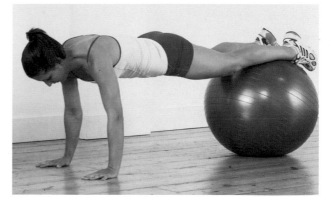

seated bicep curls, leg extended

Sets: 2
Repetitions: 12–15
Areas Worked: Front of upper arm and core

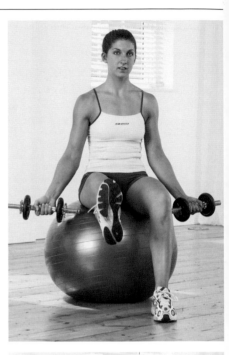

1 Sit on the ball with your feet flat on the floor.
2 Take hold of a weight in both hands with an under-hand grip, positioning them down by your side.
3 Extend one leg off the floor.
4 Flex your arms at the elbows, lifting the weights toward your shoulders.
5 Pause, and then extend your arms, lowering the weights back down to the start position.
6 Repeat, using your other leg.

Technique

- Position yourself on the center of the Swiss Ball.
- Bend one knee to 90 degrees with your foot on the floor.
- Hold your extended leg off the floor for the duration of the exercise.
- Activate and tighten your abdominal muscles, holding your back straight.
- Keep your eyes fixed straight ahead so that your neck and back are neutrally aligned.
- Hold the weights straight as you flex and extend your arms.
- Ensure that your upper arms stay vertical throughout the movement.

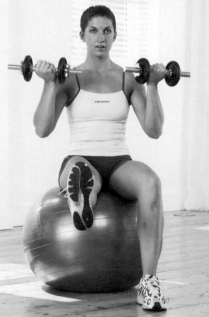

reverse bridge single leg extension

Sets: 2
Repetitions: 12–15
Areas Worked: Front of upper leg and core

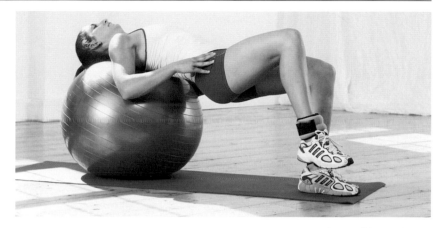

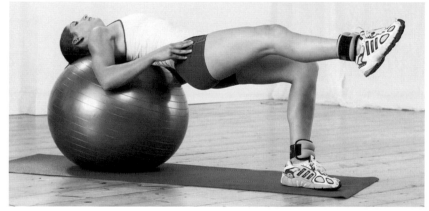

Technique

- The ball should be positioned so that it sits directly between your shoulder blades.
- Activate and tighten your abdominal muscles to help maintain a neutral alignment.
- Stabilize your weight with the foot that is on the floor.
- Keep your upper leg static and horizontal as you extend and flex your knee.
- Stop at the bottom of the movement when your knee reaches a 90-degree angle.

1 Attach an ankle weight around each ankle.

2 Lie on your back on top of the ball in the reverse bridge position, with your knees bent at 90 degrees and your right foot elevated off the floor slightly.

3 Extend your right knee, lifting your foot until your leg is straight.

4 Pause, and then flex your knee, lowering your foot back down toward the floor.

5 Repeat the exercise using your left leg.

bridge

Sets: 2
Repetitions: 10–12
Areas Worked: Buttocks, back of upper legs, and core

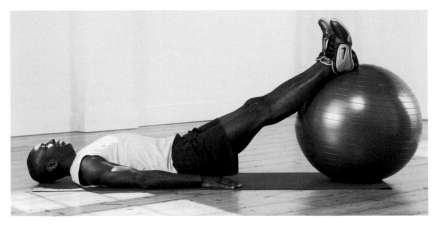

1 Position yourself lying on your back on the floor, with your heels resting on top of the ball.

2 Extend your hips, lifting your bottom off the floor.

3 Hold at the top of the movement for 3 seconds, and then flex your hips, dropping your bottom back down toward the floor.

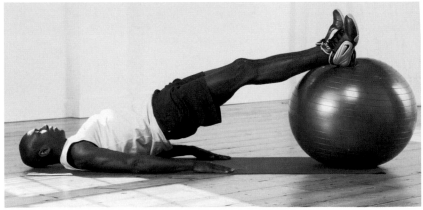

Technique

- Start with your feet on the ball and your bottom just off the floor, so that you are not resting your full weight down on the floor.
- Lift your pelvis up by extending your hips so that only the backs of your shoulders are in contact with the floor.
- Activate and tighten your core muscles to maintain the neutral position, with a straight line from your shoulders to your hips.
- Make sure that your back doesn't arch during the exercise.

sitting on the ball

Sets: 2
Time: As long as you can, or up to 1 minute
Area Worked: Core

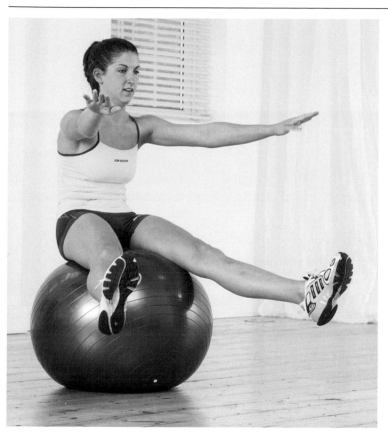

1 Sit on the ball with your feet flat on the floor.

2 Extend your arms and legs forward.

3 Hold and balance for 10 second intervals.

Technique

• Place yourself directly in the center of the Swiss Ball.

• Activate and tighten your abdominal muscles.

• Keep your eyes fixed straight ahead so that your neck and back are neutrally aligned.

• Extend your arms and legs straight so that they are not in contact with the floor.

Total Body Strength and Tone Routine—*Beginner*

chest press

Sets: 2
Repetitions: 12–15
Areas Worked: Chest, front of shoulder, back of upper arm. It also activates the muscles of the core for stability of the mid section.

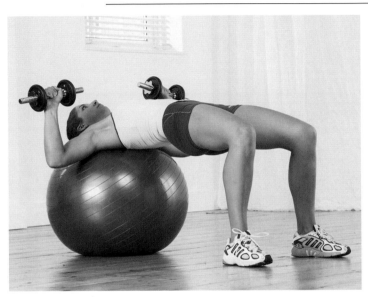

1 Lie on your back on top of the ball in the reverse bridge position, with your knees bent at 90 degrees.

2 Take hold of a dumbbell in each hand with an over-hand grip.

3 Bend elbows to 90 degrees and position them out level with your shoulders.

4 Extend both arms up, pushing the weights away, until they are straight.

5 Pause and then slowly bend arms, allowing them to return to the start position.

Technique

- The ball should be positioned so that it sits directly between your shoulder blades.
- Place feet shoulder width apart.
- Activate and tighten your abdominal muscles to help maintain a neutral alignment.
- Be careful not to let your pelvis drop and move out of alignment. You should form a straight line from shoulders through to knees.
- Ensure that forearms maintain a vertical position throughout the movement.
- Stop at the bottom of the movement when you feel a stretch across your chest and shoulders.

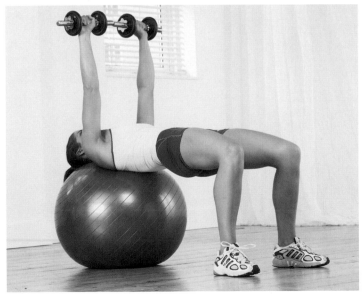

mid row

Sets: 2
Repetitions: 12–15
Areas Worked: Upper back, between shoulder blades, back of shoulders, and front of upper arms

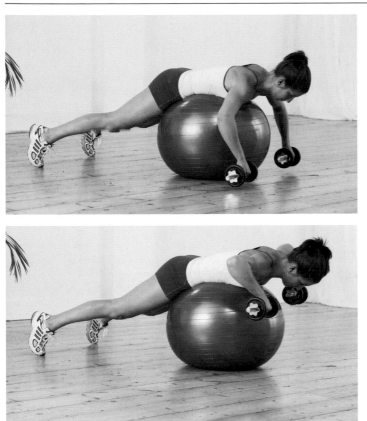

1 Position yourself lying prone on the Swiss Ball, with legs stretched out and toes on the floor.

2 Start with your upper arms out to the side and extended down toward the floor, taking hold of the weights with an over-hand grip.

3 Lift elbows up past shoulder level, bending your arms.

4 Pause, and then extend your arms, returning the weights back toward the floor.

Technique

- Your elbows should move out to the side at a 90-degree angle as you flex your arms.
- Stop at the bottom of the movement, making sure that the weights don't touch the floor.
- Ensure that your forearms are vertically positioned throughout the exercise.
- Keep your torso still during the movement.
- Make sure that your shoulders do not lift away from the ball as you raise your elbows.

seated shoulder press

Sets: 2
Repetitions: 12–15
Areas Worked: Front of shoulders and back of upper arms

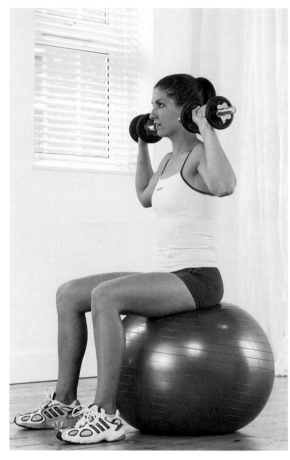
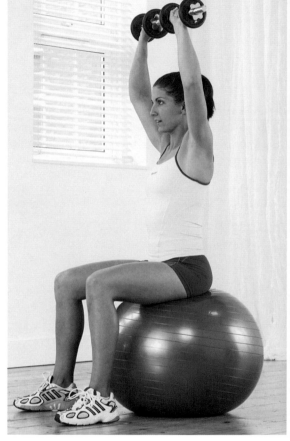

1 Sit on the ball with feet flat on the floor.

2 Take hold of a weight in both hands with an over-hand grip, positioning them just above shoulder level.

3 Extend your arms, pushing the weights above your head.

4 Pause, and then flex your arms, lowering the weights back down to the starting position.

Technique

- Place yourself directly in the center of the Swiss Ball.
- Knees should be bent to 90 degrees.
- Activate and tighten abdominal muscles.
- Keep your eyes fixed straight ahead so that your neck and back are neutrally aligned.
- Start with your elbows pointed out to the side, keeping forearms vertical.
- Extend your arms straight up so that they are vertical when fully extended.

seated bicep curls

Sets: 2
Repetitions: 12–15
Area Worked: Front of upper arm

1 Sit on the ball with feet flat on the floor.

2 Take hold of a weight in both hands with an under-hand grip, positioning them down by your side.

3 Flex your arms at the elbows, lifting the weights toward your shoulders.

4 Pause, and then extend your arms, lowering the weights back down to the starting position.

Technique

- Position yourself on the center of the Swiss Ball.
- Bend your knees to 90 degrees.
- Activate and tighten abdominal muscles, holding your back straight.
- Keep your eyes fixed straight ahead, so that your neck and back are neutrally aligned.
- Hold the weights straight as you flex and extend your arms.
- Ensure that your upper arms stay vertical throughout the movement.

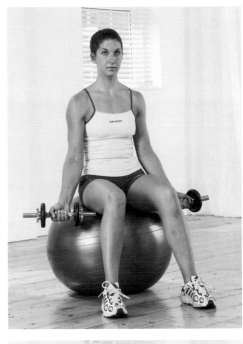

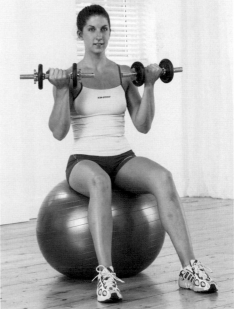

squat against wall

Sets: 2
Repetitions: 12–15
Areas Worked: Front of upper legs and buttocks

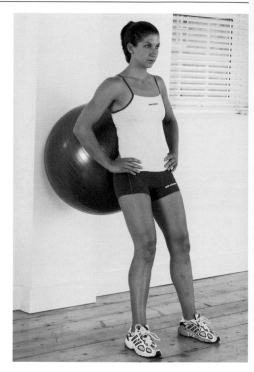

1 Place the Swiss Ball against the wall and lean your lower back into it.

2 Stand with feet shoulder width apart.

3 Flex your hips and your knees, lowering your buttocks down toward the floor, and rolling the ball up your back.

4 Pause and then extend your hips and knees, lifting yourself straight and back to the start position.

Technique

- Start with your legs straight, feet placed ahead of the ball and parallel to each other, back neutrally aligned, as you rest against the ball.
- Activate and tighten your abdominal muscles, tilting pelvis forward slightly to help maintain a neutral alignment as you flex your hips and knees.
- Look straight ahead and keep your shoulders back as you lower yourself down.
- Stop at the bottom of the movement, just before your knees reach a 90-degree angle.
- Keep your back in contact with the ball throughout the exercise.

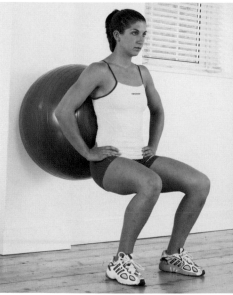

prone hamstring curls

Sets: 2
Repetitions: 12–15
Area Worked: Back of upper legs

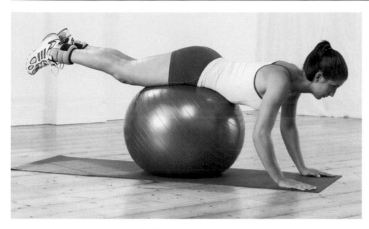

1 Secure an ankle weight around each
   ankle.

2 Lie prone on the Swiss Ball with arms
   extended, hands on the floor, and leg
   extended straight.

3 Flex your knees, lifting your feet up.

4 Pause, and then extend your legs,
   lowering your feet back down to the
   start position.

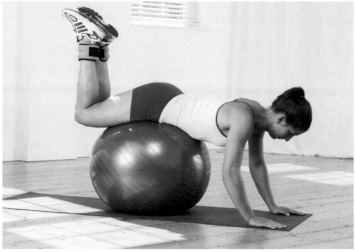

Technique

- Lie on the ball with your hips resting on the center.
- Position your hands on the floor so that they are directly below
  your shoulders.
- Hold a neutral position with a straight line running from your
  shoulders to your knees.
- Make sure that your back doesn't arch and your hips don't flex
  during the exercise.
- Keep your knees and feet together as you flex your knees.
- Flex your knees from straight legs to a 90-degree angle.

131

abdominal crunch basic

Sets: 2
Repetitions: 15–20
Area Worked: Abdomen

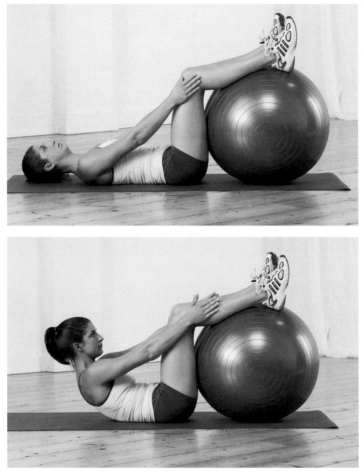

1 Position yourself lying on your back on the floor, with legs flexed and heels resting on top of the ball.

2 Roll your shoulders forward, lifting them off the floor.

3 Hold at the top of the movement for 3 seconds, and then relax back down toward the floor.

Technique

- Start with your legs flexed to 90 degrees and feet on the ball.
- Extend arms, positioning your hands on the outside of each knee.
- Activate and tighten your abdominal muscles to roll and lift your shoulders forward as you reach your hands toward your ankles.
- Make sure that only your shoulders lift away from the floor, and not your back.

back extension with toes on floor

Sets: 2
Repetitions: 12–15
Areas Worked: Lower back and sides of midsection

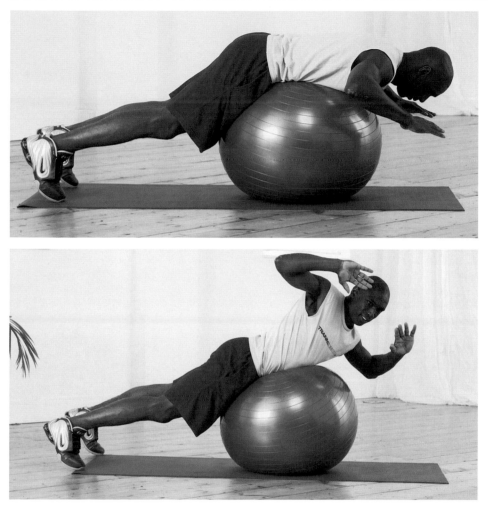

1 Lie prone on the Swiss Ball, so that your navel is on the center of the ball, with legs extended.

2 Extend your back, lifting your chest away from the ball, and rotate your torso to the right.

3 Pause, and then lower your chest and shoulders back down to the ball and starting position.

4 Repeat, extending your back and rotating your torso to the left.

Technique

- Keep your legs extended straight behind you, with toes on the floor.
- Hold arms out at a 90-degree angle to your body with your elbows bent.
- As you extend your back, slowly rotate your torso so that you are looking out to the side.
- Keep your hips square on the ball as you rotate.

Midsection Stability, Strength, and Tone Routine—*Beginner*

abdominal curl on ball

Sets: 2
Repetitions: 12–15
Area Worked: Abdomen

1 Lie on the Swiss Ball, with your knees bent at 90 degrees.

2 Extend your arms, with your hands on top of your thighs.

3 Raise your shoulders away from the ball.

4 Hold for 3 seconds and then slowly lower your shoulders back to the start position.

Technique

- Position yourself so that your mid back and upper pelvis are resting against the ball.
- Place your feet shoulder width apart.
- Drop your pelvis down slightly so that it is pressing into the ball as you raise your shoulders.
- Activate and tighten your abdominal muscles, to flex your midsection and lift your shoulders forward, as you reach your hands toward your knees.
- Stop at the bottom of the movement, just before your shoulders touch down on the ball.

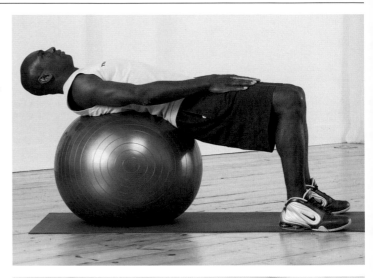

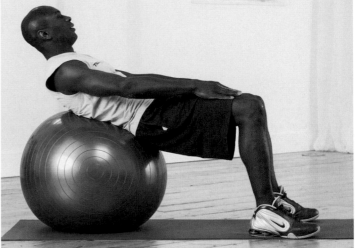

abdominal curl rotation

Sets: 2
Repetitions: 12–15
Areas Worked: Abdomen and sides of midsection

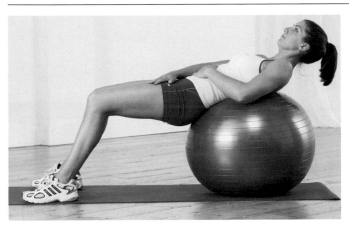

1 Lie on the Swiss Ball, with your knees bent at 90 degrees.

2 Extend your right arm, with your hand on top of your left thigh.

3 Reach your right arm along your thigh and raise and rotate your upper body and shoulders toward the left and away from the ball.

4 Hold for 3 seconds and then slowly lower yourself down, straightening your shoulders back to the start position.

5 Repeat, using your left arm and rotating toward the right.

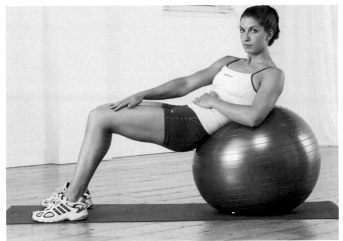

Technique

- Position yourself so that your mid back and upper pelvis are resting against the ball.
- Place your feet shoulder width apart.
- Drop your pelvis down slightly so that it is pressing into the ball as you raise your shoulders.
- Activate and tighten your abdominal muscles to flex and rotate your midsection and lift your shoulder forward as you reach your hand toward your knee.
- Stop at the bottom of the movement just before your shoulders touch down on the ball.

135

reverse curl

Sets: 2
Repetitions: 12–15
Area Worked: Lower abdomen

1 Position yourself lying on your back on the floor with your knees bent and feet raised.

2 Place the ball between your legs.

3 Flex your abdomen, tilting and lifting your pelvis off the floor.

4 Hold for 3 seconds and then lower your pelvis back down.

Technique

- Lie with your back flat on the floor.
- Position the ball between your legs, flexed to a 90-degree angle, so that the ball is in contact with your knees and lower legs.
- Make sure that your back doesn't arch or lift during the exercise.

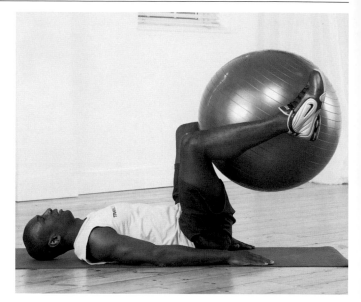

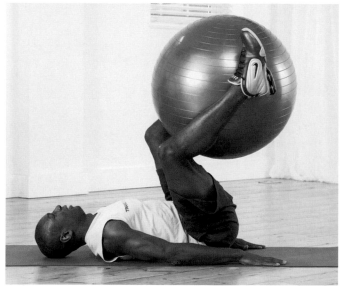

lying lateral flexion

Sets: 2
Repetitions: 12–15
Area Worked: Sides of midsection

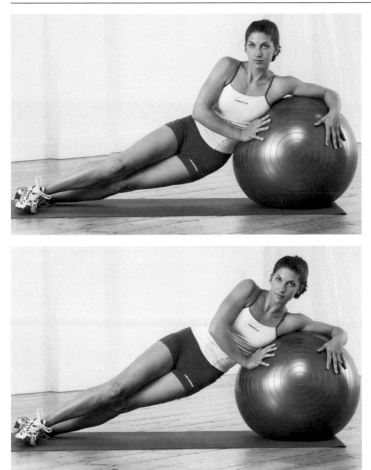

1 Lie on your left-hand side against the Swiss Ball, legs extended and feet on the floor.

2 Laterally flex your midsection, lifting your pelvis away from the floor.

3 Pause, and slowly lower your pelvis, returning back to the start position.

Technique

- Position yourself against the ball so that it is in contact with the side of your rib cage.
- Your legs should be straight, with your feet staggered.
- Bend both arms, resting one over the ball and the other on the side.
- Start with your midsection flexed toward the floor.
- Lift your pelvis away from the floor as you flex, until your body and legs form a straight line.
- Activate and tighten your abdominal muscles to help maintain a neutral back position.

reverse bridge torso rotation

Sets: 2
Repetitions: 12–15
Areas Worked: Sides of midsection and core

1 Lie on your back on top of the ball in the reverse bridge position, with your knees bent at 90 degrees.

2 Take hold of the medicine ball with both hands, and position your arms straight up.

3 Rotate your upper body to the right, rolling onto your shoulder on top of the ball.

4 Pause, and then slowly roll back with the Swiss Ball in the center of your shoulders.

5 Repeat the exercise, rotating your torso and rolling on your shoulder the other way.

Technique

- Start with the ball positioned so that it sits directly between your shoulder blades.
- Place your feet shoulder width apart.
- Activate and tighten your abdominal muscles to help maintain a neutral alignment.
- Form a straight line from shoulders through to your knees.
- Hold onto the medicine ball with your arms up, so that they are vertical, and level with your shoulders.
- Keep your arms straight throughout the movement, arcing the ball over as you roll onto your shoulder.
- Rotate your torso, rolling onto the side of your shoulder, so that it is placed in the middle of the ball.

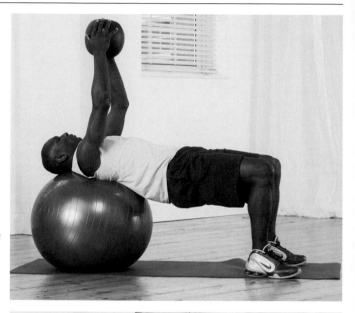

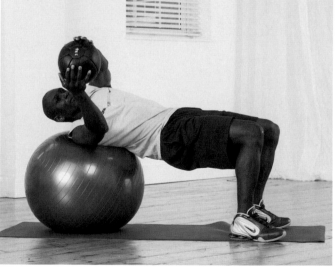

alternate arm and leg back extensions

Sets: 2
Repetitions: 12–15
Area Worked: Length of back

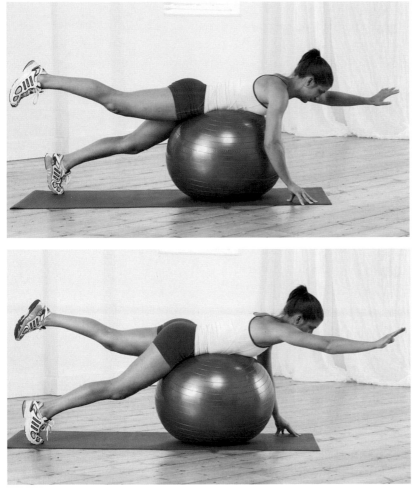

1 Lie face down on the Swiss Ball with your arms and legs extended.

2 Extend your back, lifting your left arm and right leg off the floor.

3 Hold for 3 seconds, and then lower your arm and leg back to the floor.

4 Repeat the exercise with your right arm and left leg.

Technique

- Place the opposite hand and toe on the floor to those that are elevated.
- Keep your arms and legs straight when both lifting and when static.
- Position your head so that you are facing the floor.

Total Body Stability Routine
Advanced
press ups, toes on the ball

Sets: 2
Repetitions: 12–15
Areas Worked: Chest, front of shoulders, back of upper arms, and core

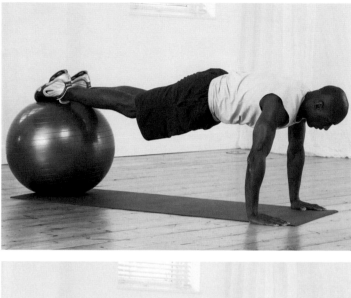

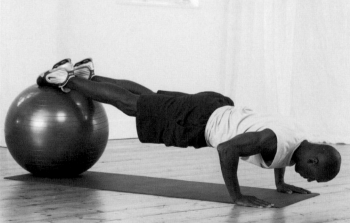

1 Position yourself on your hands with your arms extended and your toes resting on top of the ball.

2 Bend your arms, bringing your chest toward the floor until your elbows reach 90 degrees.

3 Pause, and then extend your arms, pushing your chest away from the floor, returning to the start position.

Technique

- Position your hands on the floor so that they are directly below your shoulders.
- Activate and tighten your core muscles to maintain a neutral position with a straight line running from your shoulders to your ankles.
- Make sure that your back doesn't arch during the exercise.
- Face the floor throughout the movement to keep your neck neutrally aligned.
- Your elbows should move out to the side as you bend your arms.
- Avoid locking your elbows when your arms are straight.

latissimus ball roll

Sets: 2
Repetitions: 12–15
Areas Worked: Side of back, back of shoulders, and core

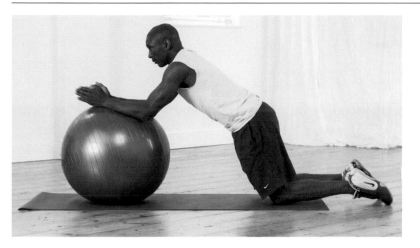

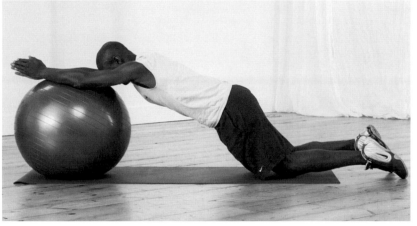

1 Kneel on the floor leaning forward, with your arms bent to 90 degrees, and rest your forearms on top of the Swiss Ball.

2 Slowly extend your arms forward, lowering your shoulders as you roll the ball away.

3 Hold the position for a few seconds, and then pull your elbows back, rolling the ball back and raising your shoulders, until you reach the start position.

Technique

- Activate and tighten your abdominal muscles to help maintain a neutral back position.
- Pivot on your knees as you lower and raise your shoulders, fixing your hips in position.
- Your elbows should end up resting on top of the ball when your arms are fully extended.
- Stop at the bottom of the movement, when you feel a stretch under your shoulders and down the side of your upper back.

kneeling shoulder press

Sets: 2
Repetitions: 12–15
Areas Worked: Front of shoulders, back of upper arms, and core

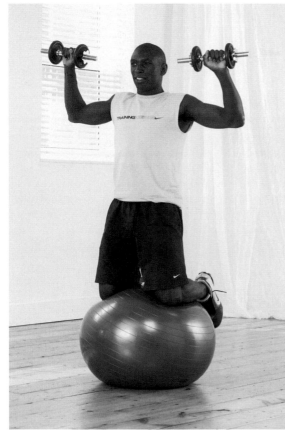 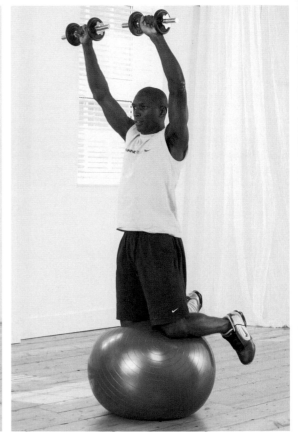

1 Take hold of a weight in both hands with an over-hand grip.

2 Kneel on top of the ball.

3 Position the weights just above shoulder level.

4 Extend your arms, pushing the weights above your head.

5 Pause, and then flex your arms, lowering the weights back down to the start position.

Technique

- Place yourself directly in the center of the Swiss Ball.
- Your knees should be bent to 90 degrees.
- Activate and tighten your abdominal muscles as you straighten your back.
- Keep your eyes fixed straight ahead so that your neck and back are neutrally aligned.
- Start with your elbows pointed out to the side, keeping your forearms vertical.
- Extend your arms straight up so that they are vertical when fully extended.

single leg squat on ball

Sets: 2
Repetitions: 12–15
Areas Worked: Front of upper legs, buttocks, and core

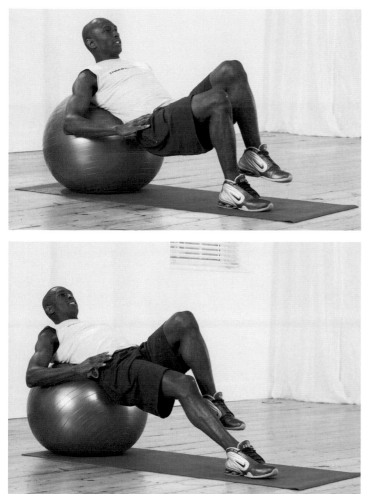

1 Lie on your back against the Swiss Ball, with your right knee bent to 90 degrees and your foot on the floor.

2 Drop your hips down until your torso is at a 45-degree angle.

3 Bend your left leg and flex your hip, holding your foot off the floor.

4 Extend your left hip and knee, rolling yourself up on the ball.

5 Pause and then flex your hip and knee lowering your bottom down toward the floor and back to the start position.

6 Repeat, using your left leg with your right foot off the floor.

Technique

- Activate and tighten your abdominal muscles to help maintain your balance as you extend your hip and knee.
- Form a straight line from your ankle to your shoulder when your leg and hip are fully extended.
- Look straight ahead and keep your shoulders back as you lower yourself down.
- Stop at the bottom of the movement, just before your knee reaches a 90-degree angle.

single leg hamstring curls

Sets: 2
Repetitions: 12–15
Areas Worked: Back of upper leg and core

1 Position yourself, lying on your back on the floor, with your right heel resting on top of the ball, and your left leg elevated.

2 Extend your hips so that you are in the reverse bridge position and hold.

3 Flex your right knee, pulling your heel toward your buttocks.

4 Pause, and then extend your right knee, dropping it down and straightening your leg back to the start position.

5 Repeat the exercise with your left heel on the ball and your right leg elevated.

Technique

- Start in the bridge position, forming a straight line from your shoulders to your ankle. Only the backs of your shoulders should be in contact with the floor.
- Activate and tighten your core muscles to maintain the neutral position.
- Make sure that your back doesn't arch during the exercise.
- Hold the inactive leg straight and above the ball so that it doesn't make contact with it.
- Flex the knee of your active leg until it is at a 90-degree angle. In this position you should be maintaining a straight line from your shoulders to your knee.

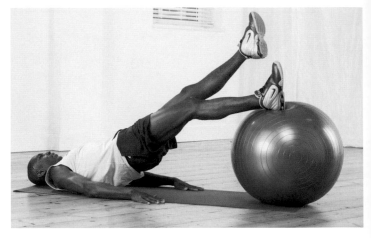

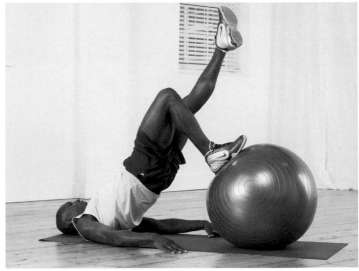

transverse abs

Sets: 2
Time: 35 seconds, or for as long as you can
Area Worked: Core

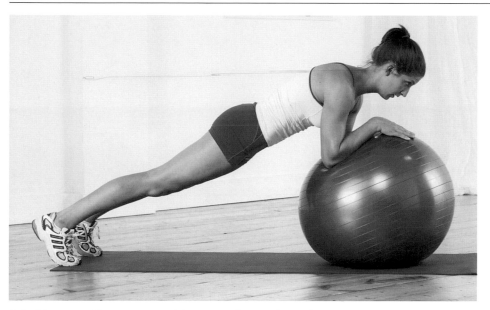

1 Position yourself on your toes with your arm bent and your forearms resting on top of the ball.

2 Hold a straight line from your ankles to your shoulders.

3 Maintain this position for as long as you can.

Technique

- Position your shoulders over your elbows so that they are vertical.
- Activate and tighten your core muscles to maintain a neutral position with a straight line running from your shoulders to your ankles.

kneeling wood chop

Sets: 2
Repetitions: 12–15
Area Worked: Core

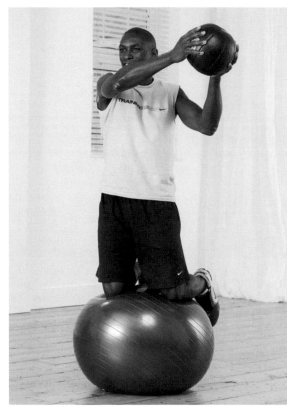 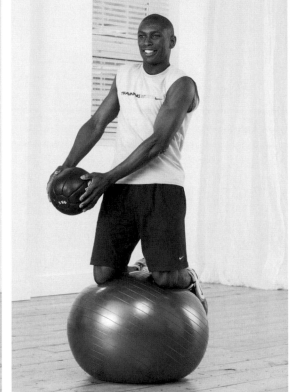

1 Kneel on the Swiss Ball, holding onto a medicine ball.

2 Start with the ball raised up and above your left shoulder.

3 Bring the ball down and across your body to the outside of the right hip.

4 Repeat, starting from your right shoulder, to your left hip.

Technique

- Position yourself kneeling on the center of the Swiss Ball.
- Activate and tighten your abdominal muscles, holding your back straight and stabilizing yourself on the ball.
- Keep your eyes fixed straight ahead so that your neck and back are neutrally aligned.
- Start by holding the ball above a shoulder with the arm that is across your body angled at 45 degrees to the opposite shoulder.
- Lower the ball down, following the 45-degree angle and extending your arms until the medicine ball reaches the outside of your opposite hip.

Total Body Strength and Tone Routine—*Advanced*
single arm chest press

Sets: 2
Repetitions: 10–12
Areas Worked: Chest, front of shoulder, back of upper arm, and the core

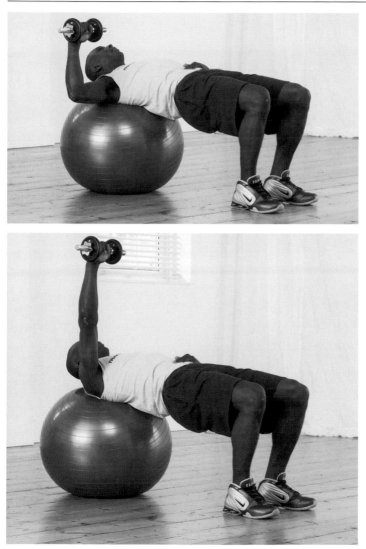

1 Lie on your back on top of the ball in the reverse bridge position, with your knees bent at 90 degrees.

2 Take hold of a dumbbell in one hand.

3 Bend your elbow to 90 degrees and position it out level with your shoulders.

4 Extend your arm up, pushing the weight away, until it is straight.

5 Pause, and then slowly bend your arm allowing it to return to the start position.

6 Continue for the desired number of repetitions and then repeat this action using your other arm.

Technique

• Position yourself on the ball so that it sits directly between your shoulder blades.

• Place feet hip width apart.

• Activate and tighten your abdominal muscles to help maintain a neutral alignment.

• Be careful not to let your pelvis drop and move out of alignment.

• Ensure that your forearm maintains a vertical position throughout each movement and whilst static.

• Rest your other hand on your stomach.

• Stop at the bottom of the movement when you feel a stretch across your chest and shoulder.

bent over single arm row

Sets: 2

Repetitions: 10–12

Areas Worked: Upper back, between shoulder blades, back of shoulder, and front of upper arm

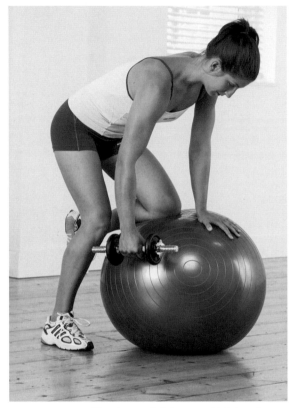 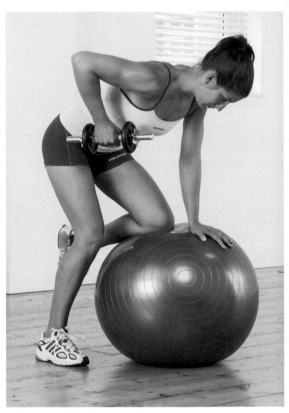

1 Position yourself with your left knee and left hand on the Swiss Ball, and right foot flat on the floor.

2 Take hold of a weight with your right hand using a palms-in grip.

3 Start with your right arm extended down toward the floor.

4 Flex your arm, lifting your elbow up and past shoulder level.

5 Pause, and then extend your arm, returning the weight back toward the floor.

6 Repeat with your left arm, placing your right hand and knee on the ball.

Technique

- Neutrally align your back and neck, fixing them in that position.
- Start with your arm straight and vertical.
- Position your elbow tight to your body as you bring the weight up, with your forearm vertical.
- Hold shoulders and hips parallel to the floor throughout the exercise.
- Keep your torso still during the movement.

single arm prone lateral raise

Sets: 2
Repetitions: 10–12
Area Worked: Back of shoulder

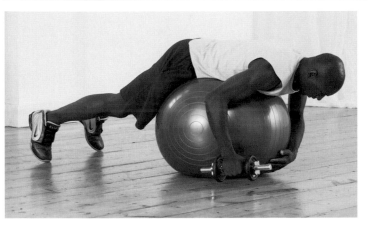

1 Position yourself lying prone on the Swiss Ball, with legs stretched out and toes on the floor.

2 Take hold of the weight in one hand with a palms-in grip.

3 Start with your arm out to the side and extended down toward the floor with a slight bend in the elbow.

4 Lift your elbow up past shoulder level, keeping your arm fixed in position.

5 Pause, and then lower your arm, returning the weight back toward the floor.

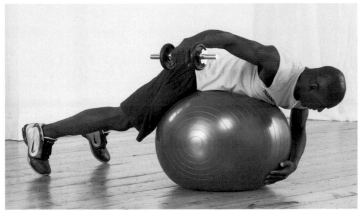

Technique

- Hold your arm in the slightly bent position throughout the exercise.
- Lift your elbow as high as you can toward shoulder height.
- The hand of your weighted arm should remain in line with your shoulder at all times.
- Stop at the bottom of the movement, making sure that the weight doesn't touch the floor.
- Keep your torso still during the movement.
- Make sure that your shoulder does not lift away from the ball as you raise your arm out to the side.

149

bicep preacher curls

Sets: 2
Repetitions: 10–12
Area Worked: Front of upper arm

1 Kneel down on the floor, leaning against the Swiss Ball.

2 Take hold of a weight in both hands with an under-hand grip, arms extended and elbows resting against the ball.

3 Flex your arms at the elbows, lifting the weights toward your shoulders.

4 Pause, and then extend your arms, lowering the weights back down to the starting position.

Technique

- Position yourself with hips pressed into the ball.
- Activate and tighten abdominal muscles, holding your back straight and shoulders high.
- Start with your arms straight and palms facing upward.
- Hold the weights straight as you flex your arms.
- Ensure that your upper arms stay fixed in position throughout the movement.

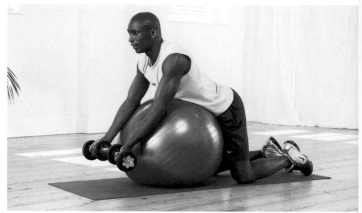

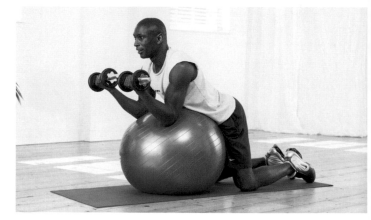

tricep dips

Sets: 2
Repetitions: 10–12
Area Worked: Back of upper arms

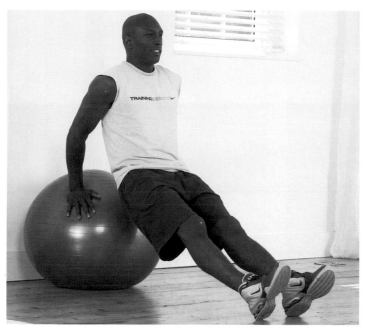

1 Place the Swiss Ball against the wall.

2 With the ball behind you, position your hands on top of it with your arms straight, and stretch out your legs in front of you so that your heels are on the floor.

3 Bend your arms, dropping your buttocks toward the floor, until elbows are at a 90-degree angle.

4 Pause, and then extend your arms, lifting yourself away from the floor and back to the starting position.

Technique

- Keep your hips flexed and legs extended throughout the movement.
- Activate and tighten your core muscles, holding your back neutrally and in a vertical position, as you flex and extend your arms.
- Pivot on your heels as you lower and raise yourself on the ball.
- Your elbows should stay parallel to each other as you bend your arms with your forearms vertical.
- Stop at the bottom of the movement when you feel a stretch across the front of your shoulders.

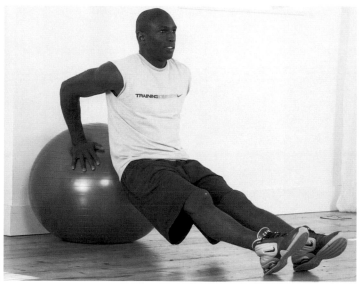

single leg squat against wall

Sets: 2
Repetitions: 10–12
Areas Worked: Front of upper legs, buttocks, and core

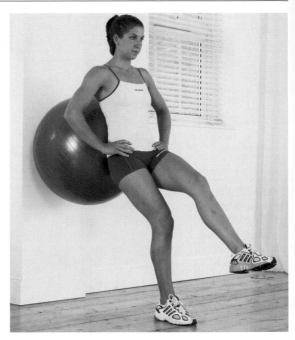

1 Place the Swiss Ball against the wall and lean your lower back into it.

2 Stand on your right leg, with left leg extended.

3 Flex your right hip and knee, lowering your buttocks down toward the floor, and rolling the ball up your back.

4 Pause, and then extend your right hip and knee, pushing yourself straight and back to the start position.

Technique

- Lean your back against the ball with your right leg straight and foot placed ahead of the ball.
- Extend your left leg and hold your foot off the floor.
- Activate and tighten your abdominal muscles, tilting your pelvis forward slightly to help maintain a neutral alignment as you flex your hip and knee.
- Look straight ahead and keep your shoulders back as you lower yourself down.
- Stop at the bottom of the movement, just before your knee reaches a 90-degree angle.
- Keep your back in contact with the ball throughout the exercise.

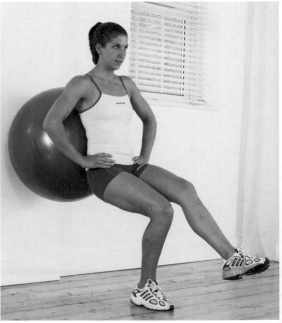

hamstring curls

Sets: 2
Repetitions: 10–12
Areas Worked: Back of upper legs and core

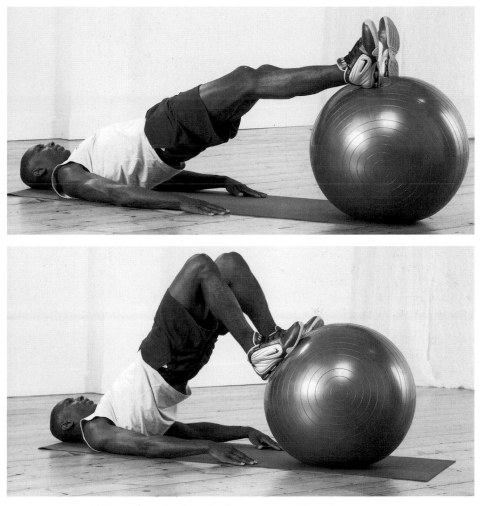

1 Position yourself lying on your back on the floor, with heel resting on top of the ball.

2 Extend your hips so that you are in the reverse bridge position and hold.

3 Flex your knees, pulling your heels toward your buttocks.

4 Pause, and then extend your knees, dropping them down and straightening your legs back to the start position.

Technique

- Start in the bridge position, forming a straight line from your shoulders to your ankles. Only the back of your shoulders should be in contact with the floor.
- Activate and tighten your core muscles.
- Make sure that your back doesn't arch during the exercise.
- Flex your knees until they are at a 90-degree angle.

153

weighted abdominal curl

Sets: 2
Repetitions: 12–15
Area Worked: Abdomen

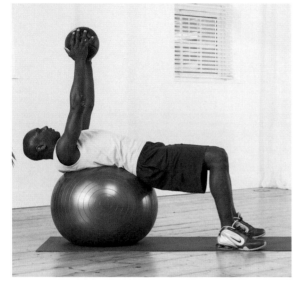 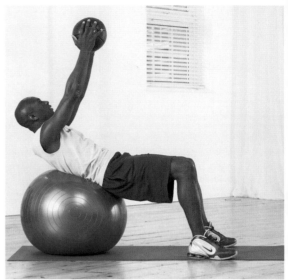

1 Lie on the Swiss Ball, with your knees bent at 90 degrees.

2 Take hold of the medicine ball and extend arms up.

3 Raise your shoulders away from the Swiss Ball.

4 Hold for 3 seconds and then slowly lower shoulders back to the start position.

Technique

- Position yourself so that your mid back and upper pelvis are resting against the ball.
- Place feet shoulder width apart.
- Drop your pelvis down slightly so that it is pressing into the ball as you raise your shoulders.
- Activate and tighten your abdominal muscles to flex your midsection and lift your shoulders forward, keeping arms and medicine ball up.
- Stop at the bottom of the movement just before your shoulders touch down on the ball.

Midsection Stability, Strength, and Tone Routine—*Advanced*

weighted abdominal curl

Sets: 3
Repetitions: 12–15
Area Worked: Abdomen

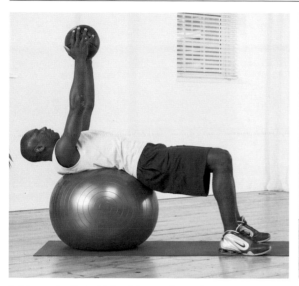 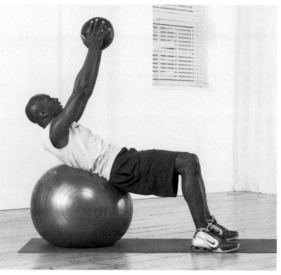

1 Lie on the Swiss Ball, with your knees bent at 90 degrees. Take hold of the medicine ball and extend your arms up.

2 Raise your shoulders away from the Swiss Ball.

3 Hold for 3 seconds and then slowly lower your shoulders back to the start position.

Technique

- Position yourself so that your mid back and upper pelvis are resting against the ball.
- Place your feet shoulder width apart.
- Drop your pelvis down slightly so that it is pressing into the ball as you raise your shoulders.
- Activate and tighten your abdominal muscles to flex your midsection and lift your shoulders forward, keeping your arms and the medicine ball up.
- Stop at the bottom of the movement, just before your shoulders touch down on the ball.

155

lying curl and flex

Sets: 3
Repetitions: 12–15
Areas Worked: Abdomen and sides of midsection

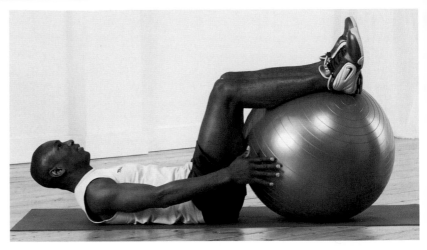

1 Position yourself lying on your back on the floor, with your knees bent and your heels resting on top of the Swiss Ball.

2 Flex your abdomen, lifting your shoulders from the floor slightly.

3 Flex your midsection, reaching your right hand down the side of the ball.

4 Pause, and then flex the other way, positioning your body straight again.

5 Repeat, flexing your midsection to the left.

Technique

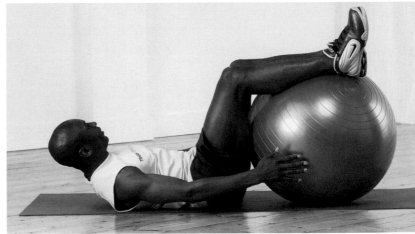

- Lie with your back flat on the floor.
- Position your lower legs with them flexed at a 90-degree angle, and so that your lower legs and heels are resting on top of the ball.
- Start with your finger tips resting on the sides of the ball, and then aim to reach them as far around the outside edge as possible.

transverse abs

Sets: 3
Time: 45 second holds
Area Worked: Core

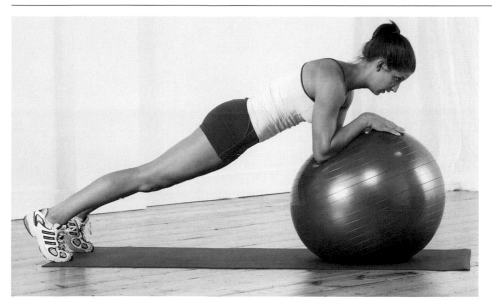

1 Position yourself on your toes with your arms bent and your forearms resting on top of the ball.

2 Hold a straight line from your ankles to your shoulders.

3 Maintain this position for as long as you can.

Technique

- Position your shoulders over your elbows so that they are vertical.
- Activate and tighten your core muscles to maintain a neutral position with a straight line running from your shoulders to your ankles.

jack knife

Sets: 3
Repetitions: 12–15
Areas Worked: Lower abdomen, front of hips, upper body, and core

1 Support yourself on your hands with your arms extended and toes resting on top of the Swiss Ball.

2 Hold a neutral position, with a straight line running from your shoulders to your ankles.

3 Flex your hips and bend your knees, pulling them in toward your body.

4 Pause, and extend your hips, taking your legs straight again, and back to the start position.

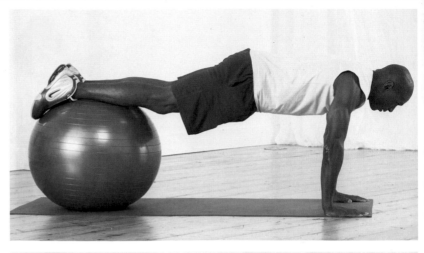

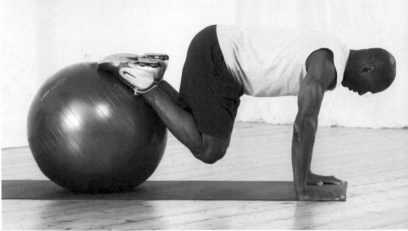

Technique

- Position your hands on the floor so that they are directly below your shoulders.
- The top of your foot and shin should be resting against the top of the ball.
- Activate and tighten your core muscles, to hold a straight line running from your shoulders to your ankles and to control your midsection, as you flex your hips.
- Flex your hips and bend your knees, pointing them toward the floor.
- Make sure that your back doesn't arch as you flex your hips.
- Face the floor throughout the movement to keep your neck neutrally aligned.

...eeling on the ball

...s: 3
...e: 45 seconds or more
...ea Worked: Core

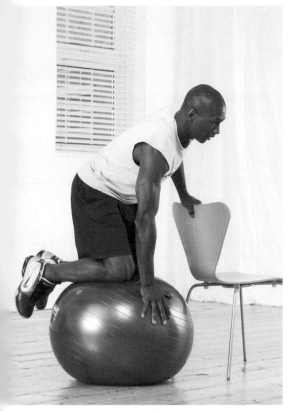

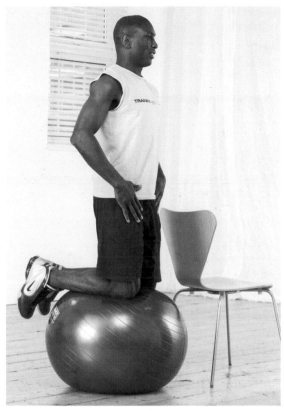

1 Stand behind the Swiss ball and place your hands and then your knees on top of the ball.

2 Slowly lift your hands away and your shoulders up until your torso is vertical.

3 Hold the position for as long as you are able to.

Technique

- Take your time in placing your hands and knees on the ball.
- Use the chair next to you to hold onto as you lift your hands away.
- Activate and tighten your abdominal muscles to help maintain a neutral back position.

Index